Natural Pregnancy

*Practical Medical Advice and
Holistic Wisdom for a Healthy
Pregnancy and Childbirth*

Lauren Feder, MD

 hatherleigh

Natural Pregnancy
Text Copyright © 2014 Lauren Feder

Library of Congress Cataloging-in-Publication Data is available.
ISBN: 978-1-57826-499-5

DISCLAIMER

This book does not give legal or medical advice. Always consult your doctor, lawyer, and other professionals. The ideas and suggestions contained in this book are not intended as a substitute for consulting with a physician. All matters regarding your health require medical supervision.

Cover and Interior Design by Carolyn Kasper

Printed in the United States

10 9 8 7 6 5 4 3 2 1

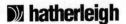

www.hatherleighpress.com

CONTENTS

VI
Natural Medicine Chest 173

DEDICATION

To Guadalupe

ACKNOWLEDGMENTS

SIMILAR TO GIVING BIRTH, writing a book is a team effort that is greatly aided by the guidance, support, and patience of others. Many thanks to my agent, Jessica Faust, and the Hatherleigh publishing team including Andrew Flach, Ryan Tumambing, Anna Krusinski, and Ryan Kennedy. In addition, my gratitude extends to the wonderful assistance and information I received from childbirth educator, Kathy Killebrew (www.imagineyourbirth.com). This all is made possible by the support of my loving family, including my dear husband, René Haarpaintner, and our wonderful children, Etienne and Quentin. We are so blessed.

—DR. LAUREN FEDER
Los Angeles, CA

Introduction to

Natural Pregnancy

THE PREGNANCY AND CHILDBIRTH experience is considered one of the most coveted experiences in a woman's life. Many women aspire for the most natural pregnancy and birth possible, yet for many this often does not come to fruition. One of the reasons is that our lives have vastly changed compared to the past: from family life, including midwifery services to the advent of modern medicine with its sophisticated technology. As a result, the diverse and vital ways in which we embrace the childbirth experience have changed. The benefits of the natural approach is that when a woman is allowed the freedom to experience her birth in her own unique way at her body's pace, undisturbed, most of the time she can have the natural birth she envisioned. This woman-centered approach—called the midwifery model of care—is beginning to gain more acceptance in hospitals where most births take place. This approach empowers the woman and in doing so allows her to experience a more meaningful childbirth. Whether a woman has a home birth or a cesarean section, the natural approach is holistic, versatile, and universal and can be used to complement a woman's needs along any step of the pregnancy journey. In the end, this is about our babies. I believe that, the more natural our approach (one which relies on healthy lifestyle choices and use of the least interventions and medications possible), the healthier our children will be for the next generation.

Maternal health is no longer just the domain of physicians, but of expectant parents. This book aims to empower parents and give them the confidence to make the best, most-informed decisions regardless of giving birth at home, at a birth center, or in a hospital. With this information, you will be given the insight needed to have the most fulfilling experience possible.

As a mother and holistic physician, I have found myself on both sides of the medical "divide." During my pregnancies, I was often simultaneously thinking as a mother-to-be and a holistic physician. I realized my background helped me in my journey as an expectant mother. Often, my explorations took me off the beaten path, exposing me to lesser-known options. As a result, I learned much about the holistic approach for pregnancy and birth, which enhanced my own wonderful experience, and which I now share with you.

Natural Pregnancy was born from this dual consciousness—from my desire to bridge the gap between expectant parents and doctors, and to encourage both parties to think more naturally, holistically, and creatively during pregnancy and beyond. In my practice, I see hundreds of pregnant women and new parents with their newborns, all with different feelings, ideas, and expectations. Whether or not they are interested in natural birth, nearly all my patients come seeking an additional approach that honors both the body and the spirit of mother and baby. It is this well-rounded approach to health that you will find in the following pages.

My Path toward Natural Medicine...and Natural Pregnancy

Like most people I know, I was not raised with natural medicine. My mother was a devoted stay-at-home mother and my father was a renowned ear, nose, and throat surgeon and voice specialist. During my teen years I underwent two thyroid surgeries and was placed on daily medication, which I was told I would take indefinitely. While doing my residency in Los Angeles a decade later, my friends were speaking about their positive experiences with a holistic practitioner. Out of intrigue (and curiosity), I decided to go as well. Within a short period of time, I was able to discontinue my thyroid medicine altogether, and have never been on anything since. The results astounded me, and thus, I began a path of discovery in the field of holistic healing, including homeopathy, for my family and patients.

What I discovered was a vital and important way of thinking about the body—not as separate body parts and organs, but as part of a whole person, inseparable from the thoughts, emotions, and experiences that make up our personalities and histories. After becoming board certified in homeopathic medicine, I opened my office with the aim of having an old-fashioned homeopathic medical practice balanced with family life. Over the years, my practice has evolved and expanded into what is now known as The Center for Natural Family Medicine, a holistic medical clinic for children and adults. We offer homeopathy, pediatrics, gynecology, and primary care medicine for adults, as well as chiropractic care from my partner and husband. We welcome newborns and their families on a regular basis, and I enjoy the interactions with pregnant couples who come seeking optimal health choices for themselves and their children.

Have you heard your mother speak about your birth? When my mother reminisced about my birth, her eyes twinkled with maternal love. Those feelings were passed down to me. Since childhood, I have always been in awe and reverence of pregnancy. During elementary school assemblies I recall looking around and envisioning all the pregnant mothers who gave birth to all those children. Ever since I was a little child, I knew I was destined for a natural birth just as my mother had done. Along the way, I have also learned that there are times when a woman would not want to have her mother's not-so-positive birth experience. From lifestyle changes to practitioner choices, I believe it is possible to change the generational patterns too.

When I learned I was pregnant, I faced a choice: have my baby in the hospital, or plan for a home birth and use a midwife. From my medical rotations in obstetrics, I remembered the IVs, bright lights, and sterile rooms of the labor and delivery wards. This atmosphere was not appealing to me, and I felt at odds with my hopes for a natural delivery. I began to explore the possibility of delivering with a midwife. A few years before, a friend had had her first child at home with a midwife and I recalled my incredulity. *What about the pain? What if there is a medical problem?* Now I found myself pregnant, and saw the option of home birth entirely differently. Rather than a sterile and impersonal environment, I could deliver my baby in my own home, supported by people who knew me well. Not familiar with midwives, I did my research. I discovered that in addition to delivering babies, midwives are experienced clinicians who provide excellent prenatal care, and are trained to handle emergencies during birth. While interviewing midwives, the offices I visited were professional, warm, and comfortable, and I felt for the first time that I was being listened to as an individual rather than just a number in a busy clinic. From my experience, the midwifery model of care's approach helps foster a viewpoint that normalizes pregnancy and has helped to legitimize the concept of a natural birth. More and more women, like myself, are seeing it as a safe choice.

As I prepared for my home birth, I began to explore the various aspects of natural parenting: making the decision between a crib versus the family bed, whether to circumcise, and if (and when) to vaccinate. Many of these alternative views on parenting were strange to my Western upbringing, but I was attracted to the "back to basics" approach. If certain ways of pregnancy and parenting had worked for generations, why fix them? And if simpler methods, such as keeping my baby in the family bed, gave me more energy to parent and resulted in a happier baby, I could see no reason to complicate my approach.

My Births

My first child, Etienne, was born in 1993, and I remember this event as if it were yesterday, because the birth of our babies marks one of the most special days in our lives as women. Never having had any ultrasounds, it was wonderful to look forward to finding out whether my baby was a girl or a boy, the old-fashioned way. According to my dates, I delivered thirteen days past my due date, not uncommon for a first baby. One of my husband René's roles was kitchen duty, heating up water which the midwife used to make warm compresses with small towels (placed on the perineum). Switching between a low tone or hum, I vocalized my way through my contractions, sometimes even falling asleep in between them. With a first labor of 13 hours, including several hours of pushing, my baby was born. My midwife said, "Lauren, you can lift your baby out now." In a surreal way, I placed this luscious warm being on my chest. Surrounded by my family and friends, Etienne came into this world.

Quentin's birth in 1997 was completely different, of course. I always tell my patients that if one child is "night" than the other is usually "day." A few days before my due date, I noticed the slightest trickle before going to bed. I called my midwife and we decided it was probably that my water had broken, but ever so slightly. Not experiencing any contractions or rise in temperature (which she asked me to check, following standard procedure when the waters break to make sure there is not an infection) she encouraged me to go to sleep. Excited and in anticipation that I would be going into labor and having a baby, it was hard to fall asleep, needless to say. The next day I took long walks, but nothing happened, except the occasional trickle. In contact with my midwife, we made an appointment for the following day. Sometime during the second night, I woke up from dreams that I was having cramps—which I was. Compared to my first labor in which I was relatively sedentary, my second one was "on the run." My body knew how to birth and proceeded to move at a lightning pace that I called "fast and furious." With each contraction I was either in a different position, different room or on the toilet. I credit my husband, as well as my cold, wet washcloth which I rubbed on my tummy and face, with helping me through the contractions. It all happened so quickly; the midwife arrived, and with a few pushes Quentin was born ten minutes later in the wee hours of the morning. I will never forget Etienne, then four years old, waking up to find that he had a new brother.

My births were uneventful from the midwife's viewpoint. If I had been within the hospital setting, I might have had different experiences altogether. With my first birth I was nearly two weeks past due, and I might have needed to be induced, as some doctors do not permit women to go much past their due dates. For my second birth, because my water had broken, most medical models expect a woman to deliver within 24 hours. However, I did not go into labor until about 27 hours later. I am grateful for my experiences, which empowered me as a woman who wanted to experience a meaningful childbirth and felt I had received the gold standard in maternity care.

My experiences in pregnancy, during birth, and after birth were superb, and I have made it one of my priorities to educate people about lesser-known options to standard delivery. But whether you go with home birth or the hospital, the natural approach is a philosophy that will fit to your comfort level and lifestyle. It encompasses wisdom that has been passed on through generations by mothers, fathers, healers, and midwives, and has been tried and tested in my own life and many others. Most importantly, the natural way for pregnancy, birth, and beyond is about trusting your instincts. We *know* how to be pregnant, give birth, and parent naturally, but what we are taught often contradicts our initial instincts.

All of our pregnancies are unique and special. Even though I chose to not have any ultrasounds and gave birth at home, this book seeks to meet you where you are on your journey of motherhood, and perhaps take you further. While this is a book on the natural approach to pregnancy and birth, I have also devoted many pages to the standard medical model—complete with details about interventions, procedures, and medications. I am well aware that most of us grew up with medical doctors and nurses, and for birth, many women feel more "at-home" in the hospital environment. It is my hope that the gems I have received over the years, which I present to you in this book, can be used whether you are having a homebirth or require a cesarean section. The birth tips and natural and homeopathic medicines found in these pages are universal, effective, and safe.

History Overview: The Medicalization of Childbirth

Natural pregnancy and birth are as old as time itself. For as long as we go back through humanity, women have given birth, naturally. By looking at the past we gain perspective on pregnancy and birth attitudes in the twenty-first century, as it is only recently that modern medicine has become intricately involved in the birth process.

Historically, our ancestors lived in small villages where local women, mothers and midwives (translated as "*with the woman*" in Middle English), supported the woman and helped her during pregnancy and especially in birth, as well as during the postpartum period, if needed. Before the twentieth century, nearly everyone delivered at home. If a woman was too poor, she had to deliver in the hospital. In those days, hospitals were unclean places, filled with infections, where the poor went to die.

By the seventeenth century, pregnancy and birth became a point of interest by the emerging medical community, starting what is now coined as the "medicalization of childbirth." By the early twentieth century, most births (both normal and complicated) became *medicalized* in developed countries. Eventually, medical doctors managed the care of women during childbirth, replacing the majority of midwives. As a result of the increasing intervention and control by doctors, childbirth became viewed less as a normal, natural experience and more as a medical procedure which needed to be orchestrated with pain medications, shaving of pubic hair, and ultimately leaving women no options or choices in the matter. In the twenty-first century, most Western industrialized countries have adopted similar medical models of care. Although, outside of the United States, midwives still play a greater role in labor and delivery.

In the past, life was different too. People's lives were greatly influenced by factors such as food supplies, harvest, weather, war, and infectious diseases. As a result the mortality rate was higher in women and children compared to today. Before the twentieth century, 1 percent of women died from pregnancy-related complications and up to 25% of babies died before one year old. Due to a lack of knowledge about proper hygiene and sanitation before the twentieth century, it came to light that physicians (not midwives) were responsible for the rise in maternal mortality According to physician (and writer) Oliver Wendell Holmes, physicians who went from performing autopsies to delivering babies, spread infection (known as *puerperal fever*) from patient to patient because of dirty, infected hands.

Also at that time, the industrial revolution was in full swing leading to crowded, unclean living conditions in factories and cities. Eventually, improvements in sanitation, healthcare, literacy, nutrition, and standard of living witnessed a decrease in the infant and maternal mortality rates in the United States by over 90%. However, according to midwife Ina May Gaskin, "There has been no decline in our national maternal death rate since 1982. This is significant, since the rate of maternal death in our country declined every year between the mid-1930s and 1982." While this is true for the United States, this is not the case in other wealthy countries where there has been a decline. The reason: the U.S. medical system is complex and different from those of other industrialized countries. Gaskin, founder of the Safe Motherhood Quilt Project, is an advocate for the midwifery model of care which endorses a safe, woman-centered childbirth method. Due to the predominance of obstetricians delivering babies in U.S. hospitals, there are far fewer midwifery deliveries compared to other similar countries. Midwives, compared to obstetricians, are trained in normal vaginal births, while the latter are trained surgeons. As a result, the United States' C-section rate has increased, as have the mortality rates.

Fear and Anxiety: The Nocebo Effect

Despite this dramatic decline in mortality rates and general improvements in healthcare, the thread of fear and anxiety is still tightly woven in our society, and is especially evident in the maternity ward. In general, we live in a risk-based society where decisions are made based on fear, and the medical world is no exception. Pregnancy, and especially birth, is often treated as if they are an illness or a dangerously abnormal process. This approach only fosters the thinking that, without medical intervention in a hospital setting, it would be impossible to have a healthy baby. As opposed to being viewed as a normal natural bodily function that has occurred since the beginning of time, the simple birth process of the past has now become a complex entity, as well as a business.

From the use of ultrasounds and sophisticated genetic testing in pregnancy to that of fetal monitoring and medications used in labor, many women are reassured and appreciate having knowledge about their unborn baby. On the other hand, sometimes women become burdened with feelings of uncertainty, worry, and tentativeness by having the information. As a result, it is not surprising that anxiety levels run high during pregnancy. These negative thoughts and feelings have recently been coined the *nocebo effect*. Research findings suggest that placebo effects can work both ways. The *placebo* ("I will please" in Latin) effect is when one expects that a treatment or experience will be helpful and thereby experiences a positive result, even if given a sugar pill. Alternatively, the nocebo effect occurs when anticipation of negative effects or unnecessary worry leads to the development of symptoms even though it is not warranted. This is often fueled by the power of suggestion which can be conveyed from our healthcare practitioners, who provide their expertise along with their own thoughts, feelings, and experiences surrounding health, pregnancy, and birth. According to research, the labor and delivery nurse serves as the primary decision maker in managing a woman's labor at the hospital, which ultimately influences the birth outcome. As we place our confidence in our healthcare providers, even casual comments such as the baby's size or position, increases stress and leads to a nocebo effect with actual physical manifestations such as increased blood pressure and pulse and muscle tightness—all of which can transform a blissful pregnancy into a terrifying experience. The mere anticipation of pain, potential risks, and complications can trigger the nocebo effect, leading to a self-fulfilling prophesy. Ultimately, the nocebo effect may not be entirely avoided, but it can be less pronounced when women familiarize themselves with the choices and aptly participate with their practitioner in being a decision maker. Healthcare providers can also take care in *how* the information is presented so, when possible, they can appropriately minimize or prevent anxiety for the woman.

According to birth pioneer Dr. Michel Odent, "Pregnant women always had the intuitive knowledge that the development of their baby in the womb was influenced by their emotional state. The more aware we are of the importance of the emotional states of pregnant women, the more we take into consideration the possible "nocebo effect" of antenatal (prenatal) care." Because of this intimate patient-doctor relationship, healthcare practitioners need to be thoughtful in dealing with patients' belief systems and emotional susceptibility when discussing tests, medications, and even childbirth.

FROM THE DOCTOR'S DESK

Katy, a family doctor, visited her obstetrician in her last trimester and was told that she was "carrying" low and would probably deliver a small baby way before her due date. According to the obstetrician's experience this was a common occurrence for hardworking female physicians. Ultimately, Katy gave birth two weeks past her due date to a son who weighed 8 lb, 6 oz (3.8 kg). He was neither small nor early! Katy said that her obstetrician's comments were a source of unnecessary anxiety and worry about her baby. She confided that this nocebo effect could have been avoided if he had gently encouraged her to make sure she find a balance between work and personal time, especially in her last trimester.

Like most women, I was afraid of childbirth. Would it hurt? Would I be able to handle it? In my prenatal yoga class, one by one, each of us would graduate to becoming a mother, leaving the rest of the class with our stories, and great hopes for our futures. Whenever I felt a surge of worry for the inevitable, I would remind myself that millions of women have experienced childbirth, including generations upon generations of our ancestors. Even though this was a new experience for me, I felt empowered because my body knows what to do. I thoughtfully chose my birth team, which included my midwife, Leslie; my prenatal yoga teacher, Gurmukh; my birth teacher, Davi; and my backup physician Dr. Paul Crane, along with my husband, several friends, and my parents. Their support gave me the confidence to enter the unknown regions and trust in the wisdom of our birthright of becoming a mother.

Benefits and Risks of Modern Medicine

Despite the fact that birth is medicalized in most developed countries, the benefits of intervention have lessened the risks from complications such as placenta previa, when the placenta partially or totally covers mother's cervix, as well as ectopic pregnancy, a tubal pregnancy. (Both may lead to severe bleeding and require medical procedures.) For some women, the benefits from epidural anesthesia have allowed them to participate in their births and be fully aware, albeit without the discomfort. Yet, most routine medical interventions such as fetal monitoring, episiotomy, and lithotomy position for birthing (lying on the back with knees and feet positioned above the hips, in stirrups), can even pose increased risks, and do not necessarily have proven benefits. Moreover, many women, in spite of having delivered a healthy child, suffer from childbirth trauma due to such factors as unexpected medical intervention, feeling a lack of dignity, and limited control in decision making.

The childbirth process moves at a certain pace, which differs from birth to birth. Medical interference forces women to be passive and does not allow them to participate in their birth, thereby taking away their dignity and respect and resulting in a detached birth event. Critics of medicalized births argue that routine practices in the hospital can trigger a cascade of events that increases the chance of using medications for induction, pain, and ultimately surgery (a cesarean section). All of this comes with its set of risks. According to research from Stanford, the source of the culture of modern birth practices is *doctor-technology-centric* rather than *patient-centric*, the latter is also known as *mother-friendly*.

Mother-Friendly Care

Although I believe in the "best of both worlds" approach, and appreciate the backup medical support for emergencies, I am a fan of the more simple mother-friendly approach which recognizes, respects, and encourages the natural laws of pregnancy exquisitely designed by Mother Nature. The Mother-Friendly Childbirth Initiative was started by a group of practitioners and laypeople who were concerned that normal and natural childbirth was becoming less commonplace and this was affecting the well-being of mothers, babies and their families. In order to be designated "mother-friendly," a hospital, birth center, or home birth service must be compliant with philosophical principles surrounding birth including access to support, freedom of movement, nondrug methods of pain relief, and breastfeeding, many of which are discussed throughout this book. These programs help to promote a prevention and wellness model of maternity care while helping improve birth outcomes and reduce costs. In general, when a birth is allowed to proceed at its natural pace, most births are normal.

What Is Natural Pregnancy and Birth?

Natural childbirth implies being in accordance with the way that Mother Nature intended for women to give birth. When a laboring woman is undisturbed and uninterrupted in a private, serene, and safe environment, she will usually deliver her baby normally. Natural birth is defined as a vaginal birth free of pain medication, with minimal or no use of interventions such as forceps or episiotomy. The natural approach to pregnancy and childbirth:

- ✿ Recognizes the importance of many age-old birthing traditions that have been used successfully for generations.
- ✿ Is mother-friendly in that it reassures women that ultimately, beyond any medicine, procedure or test, pregnancy, birth, and motherhood are symbolic of empowerment, pride, and their life-giving force.
- ✿ Encourages women to trust their common sense and intuition, and partner with their practitioner in decision making when needed.
- ✿ Discourages blind faith in the standard medical profession, which is preoccupied with intervention rather than prevention.
- ✿ Meets the needs and well-being of pregnant women in a way that is as natural as possible, yet can be used alongside standard medicine when needed, without mutual exclusivity.
- ✿ Relies on natural methods and medicines that are safe, nontoxic and natural with no side effects rather than using potentially harmful medications and interventions during birth.
- ✿ Respects the ways of the human body, and patiently honors the birth process.

Why Natural Childbirth?

There are various reasons why women choose natural childbirth. For many, a natural birth experience is often described to be "'beyond words," and profoundly satisfying. To be able to tap into an intuitive wisdom is an empowering experience.

In our busy, technologically driven lives, we become detached from our feminine, maternal nature. Yet, it is amazing how easy it can be facilitated, when a woman is surrounded by a warm, loving, experienced birth team that encourages her and provides her the liberty to embrace this life-giving event. Other women desire a natural approach because they have had a negative experience with the standard medical system, often citing dissatisfaction or that they feel traumatized because of failure to offer effective, safe, or humane care. Some women choose a more natural pregnancy and birth because of concerns of possible injury or harm to the baby incurred from interventions such as ultrasound or epidurals, many of which are not acknowledged by the medical model of care (see Chapter 2). In the *Journal of Perinatal Education*, Dr. Judith Lothian writes, "...the most compelling reason to choose natural childbirth is a universal one. Women know how to give birth without machines, epidurals, and fear. Why natural childbirth? The more important question might be 'Why not.'"

Natural Medicine for Any Birth

The natural approach is a philosophy that will adapt, enhance, and facilitate every woman's pregnancy and birth. It encompasses practical wisdom that has been passed on through generations by mothers, fathers, healers, and midwives. It utilizes natural medicines such as homeopathy when needed. Most importantly, the natural path is about trusting one's instincts to find the best approach for birth. Regardless of how a woman chooses to deliver her baby, she has the possibility of having a fulfilling birth. This book will, among other things, encourage you to have confidence in your own judgment and learn for yourself.

Holistic Medicine and Homeopathy

Holistic medicine encompasses a wide variety of practices, including homeopathy, herbs, acupuncture, ayurveda, osteopathy, naturopathy, and chiropractic care. What unites these different methodologies is a common belief that bodies are more than a sum of their parts, and that medicine should account for the whole person—mind as well as body. The word holistic derives from the word, "whole," and holistic medicine takes an integrated approach to treatment, asking not only what is happening symptomatically to the body, but what emotional, psychological, or environmental factors may be contributing to the issue. Also crucial to holistic medicine is the emphasis on natural, nontoxic remedies and procedures. Holistic practitioners generally believe that the natural approach is usually a safer and more effective means of treating illness than conventional medicines, with fewer side effects and less wear and tear on the body.

In contrast to standard medicine, which generally is solely preoccupied with the physical body and its physiology, holistic medicine views health and illness as products of the spirit as much as the body. If our minds are distressed, our emotions in turmoil, and our environment toxic or stressful, our bodies will let us know. Forms of treatment like homeopathy and Chinese medicine are considered *energy medicines*, because they work not only on physical processes, but on the deeper forces that balance body, mind, and emotions. Energy medicines conceive of health as influenced by what is called the *vital force*, the fundamental animating energy in living beings. While conventional medicine tends to rely on chemical and mechanical explanations for illness, holistic practices understand illness in terms of balance. A body seeks balance, or homeostasis, but occasionally, due to a variety of factors, it is not strong enough to ward off disease. Homeopathy and other forms of natural medicine seek to restore balance by strengthening the whole person's ability to resist illness at the core level. Conventional medicine, in contrast, seeks to combat an illness by combating primarily its symptoms.

Homeopathy is a natural system of medicine that works by using a small dose of a substance to help stimulate the body's healing forces. Homeopathy is a safe treatment that is gentle yet extremely effective when used properly. In 1789, a young physician in Europe named Samuel Hahnemann made a brilliant medical discovery. He called it *homeopathy*. Although the principles date back to Hippocrates, it was Dr. Hahnemann who was credited with organizing it into a modern scientific and medical system.

News of his exciting discoveries spread quickly. By the early 1800s, homeopathic practitioners had arrived on the shores of the New World. In America, homeopathy's popularity continued to spread after American doctors had great success with it in the treatment of the cholera epidemic of 1849. In addition, many folks relied on homeopathic remedies to treat common, mild ailments at home. By 1900, there were over 100 homeopathic hospitals in the United States alone.

Homeopathy's many supporters included Britain's royal family, Louisa May Alcott, Gandhi, Harriet Beecher Stowe, Goethe, and many others. The homeopathic remedies described in this book are for basic self-limiting conditions that do not require a medical diagnosis. These are minor illnesses or conditions with few symptoms. The homeopathic treatment of severe illnesses and chronic diseases requires the expertise of a professional homeopath.

The principle of homeopathy is based on the "law of similars." In other words, minute homeopathic doses of a substance that in large amounts could cause symptoms can heal you. Let's look at an example: The homeopathic remedy *Allium cepa* (red onion) is used to treat the runny nose and watery eyes from a cold or hay fever, the very symptoms it would cause if one were cutting a red onion in the kitchen. For pregnancy-related conditions, there are hundreds of remedies that homeopathic practitioners use. From amniocentesis to labor contractions, homeopathic medicines can be used safely and effectively alongside any medication or procedure (including surgery), to allow a woman and her birth team to participate in the birthing process and to enhance the experience.

How to Use This Book:
The Midwifery Model and Homeopathic Medicines

This book is twofold. It is not meant to replace your healthcare provider, but rather to introduce you to the possibilities that lie beyond the medical model of obstetrical care (known as the midwifery model of care), and to also expand your home medicine cabinet with a multitude of simple, practical, and time-honored methods as well as homeopathic medicines (also referred to as remedies) and other natural treatments. Knowing when and how to use the remedies can help shorten the duration of complaints and conditions in pregnancy and head others off before they start. One such medicine is *Sepia*, which is a commonly used remedy for women. In my second pregnancy, I experienced bouts of mild dizziness which my midwife considered a "not-to-worry" symptom. One dose of *Sepia* cleared my head and I fully enjoyed the remainder of my pregnancy with no other complaints. *Sepia* is also an excellent remedy for morning sickness, especially with sensitivity to odors. Countless expectant mothers have benefited from taking *Sepia* for pregnancy nausea.

Many homeopathic medicines are similarly effective and versatile, and the key to using them is knowing that they are available. This introduction to *Natural Pregnancy* sets the tone by establishing a foundation of the importance of natural pregnancy. Chapter 1 gives you information on optimizing your health, while Chapter 2 introduces you to choices in birth practitioners as well as the routine tests offered during pregnancy, albeit with additional viewpoints that often are not considered. Chapter 3 covers labor basics including birth hormones, as well as natural and medical interventions. Chapter 4 offers more psychosocial information regarding roles of fathers as well as a discussion of grief and sorrow surrounding pregnancy. And all expectant parents can make use of the A to Z compendium of treatments for common conditions in pregnancy, as well as commonly used remedies during labor, found in Chapter 5.

Whether your concern is dealing with heartburn or labor preparation, this book presents the conventional approach along with the natural treatments and remedies that are easy to administer at home. Finally, Chapter 6 also includes a "Natural Medicine Chest" of common, everyday remedies, exercises, and tools safe for home use. Most basically, this book is meant to expand your healthcare options during pregnancy, and introduce you to remedies and natural solutions that I have seen make profound differences in women's lives—including my own. Ultimately, the reason we desire to be healthy during pregnancy and have a safe birth, is for the sake of our children, the next generation. Nothing matters more to us than the health of our children, but oftentimes because we have busy lives and as we are creatures of comfort, we stick to what is familiar even if we know the results may not be ideal. This book provides simple, step-by-step advice on working natural health into "regular" habits, and in the process, will also give you a means of thinking about your health (and your child's) holistically—with an abundance of vitality, joy, and curiosity.

I wish you a wonderful pregnancy and joyous birth.

—Dr. Lauren Feder

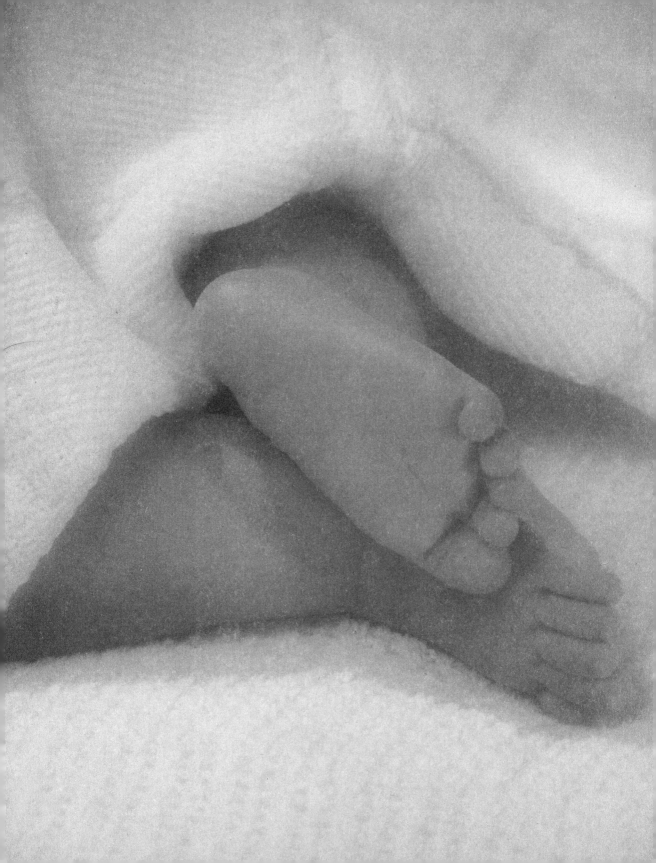

Optimizing Your Health:
Before, During, and After Pregnancy

Lifestyle Choices and Pregnancy

Healthcare practitioners are beginning to acknowledge how lifestyle factors such as nutrition, exercise, relationships, and stress during pregnancy can profoundly impact babies with lifelong effects. For this reason, pregnancy is the time when many women take the best care of themselves to ensure optimal health for their children. Ideally, preparation for baby begins with the couple, before conception, on a physical, emotional, and spiritual level. However, it is never too late to begin! From eating healthy, exercising, and seeking out harmony in your relationship and workplace, you are important in all ways. Like a bird who builds a nest or an athlete preparing for a marathon, one of the most important aspects to consider when having a child is preparation. It is said that an apple doesn't fall far from the tree, and for this reason having a healthy child begins with us. Although most women aim to take good care of themselves *during* pregnancy, I encourage you to take a holistic look at yourself—before, during, and after baby.

Nutrition and Pregnancy

It is said that food is our best medicine. For a healthy approach to eating, I focus on the work of two doctors in the area of pregnancy and nutrition (and beyond): Drs. Thomas Brewer and Weston A. Price. I appreciate Dr. Brewer's daily recommendations and suggested quantities alongside the wholesome ingredients from the Weston A. Price pantry.

The Dr. Brewer Pregnancy Diet

Dr. Brewer, who practiced in the twentieth century, is known for his emphasis on the importance of nutrition during pregnancy, a novel idea compared to many of his other colleagues at the time. "On my list of concerns about my pregnant patients' welfare, nutrition ranks second only to breathing. The reason is simple: well-nourished women develop far fewer complications in pregnancy, have more efficient labors, and give birth more easily to healthier babies than do their poorly nourished sisters. This makes my job as an obstetrician much easier—and a lot more enjoyable!" His goal was to keep his patients healthy in their pregnancies, and he believed that such conditions as preeclampsia (toxemia) marked by high blood pressure, high levels of protein in the urine, and significant swelling in hands and feet, are preventable through proper nutrition. His diet provides specific guidelines which includes calcium 1200 mg/day, 80 to100 mg protein/day, Vitamin C, and more. As my birth teacher, Kathy Killebrew said, "Don't look at the scale. When you eat healthy the weight gain will take care of itself."

The Dr. Brewer Pregnancy Diet for a Healthy Mom and Baby

(Adapted from *Right from the Start* by Gail Brewer)

Every day of the week, you and your baby must have:

- Milk and milk products (4 choices): milk, yogurt, cottage cheese, cheese
- Calcium replacements: almonds, broccoli, blackstrap molasses, kale
- Eggs (2)
- Protein combinations (6–8 choices): chicken, fish, salmon, brewer's yeast, beans and rice
- Fresh, dark green vegetables (2 choices): collard greens, asparagus, broccoli, spinach
- Whole grains (5 choices): oatmeal, brown rice, granola, whole grain bread
- Foods containing Vitamin C (2 choices): orange, strawberries, green pepper, potato
- Fats and oils (3 choices): butter, avocado, peanut butter
- Foods containing Vitamin A (1 choice): carrots, sweet potato, apricots, pumpkin
- Liver once a week (optional)
- Salt and other sodium sources (to taste): sea salt, kelp powder, soy sauce
- Water (unlimited)
- Snacks and additional menu choices (from food groups listed above)
- Optional supplements: vitamins, molasses, etc.

For more information, go to Dr. Brewer's Pregnancy Diet at www.drbrewerpregnancydiet.com. This site also includes substitutes for meat and dairy, and for women with food allergies.

Sacred Foods for the Next Generation

Going beyond the standard dietary recommendations lies a vast area of information and research that has led me to rethink the concept of healthy nutrition based on the work of Dr. Weston A. Price, an American dentist from the 1930s. In his quest to discover reasons for tooth decay, Dr. Price travelled the world and studied groups of isolated communities worldwide who enjoyed excellent dental health. Although the non-industrialized peoples he studied came from different geographical regions, they all had the following in common:

❀ Traditional diet of indigenous foods

❀ Long, healthy lives

❀ No chronic illness, obesity, infertility, or birth defects

❀ Strong bones and straight teeth (including no cavities)

Reading about Dr. Price's work struck a chord within as I have respected many of the traditional customs of our healthy ancestors. Focusing on their nutrition, he found that these groups shared common eating habits. Much to my surprise they were not vegetarians! In fact, they consumed nutrient dense foods high in vitamins and minerals such as cream, butter, eggs, organ meats, fish, fish oils, and shellfish.

In his research Dr. Price saw that each group reserved the most nutritious foods, known as "sacred foods," for the next generation which included couples in their pre-conception phase, pregnant women, nursing mothers, babies, and children. One of the staple foods of healthy ancestors was bone broths (what we know as chicken soup) which provide calcium for healthy bones and teeth. Grains and nuts were soaked, sprouted and/or fermented for easier digestion. The use of high quality butter and other animal fats were prized for health and fertility. In standard medicine, high cholesterol (and obesity) is thought to be linked to consuming a higher fat diet, hence we are encouraged to avoid foods high in fat. However, according to the Weston A Price Foundation, cholesterol plays many vital roles in the body. Fermented vegetables (such as sauerkraut or kimchi) and dairy products (kefir, yogurt) provide healthy bacteria similar to probiotics. Little by little I have implemented tasty culinary dishes with these benefits when cooking for my family. Although this diet is not vegetarian, there are many preparations that vegans will find helpful, including sauerkraut, tempeh, and sprouted nuts and seeds.

The following is a list of Weston A. Price suggestions for pregnant and nursing mothers. Ideally, these diet modifications should be started before conception:

Butter: What doesn't taste better with butter? Butter is high in Vitamin A which is needed for proper functioning of the thyroid and adrenals, and also improves growth, heart function, and protein and calcium assimilation. Also known for its anti-oxidant properties, butter contains lecithin, which aids in the metabolism of cholesterol and fat. It also has many important minerals, fatty acids, and Vitamins D, E, and K. Healthy sources of butter include raw and organic butter, as well as high vitamin butter oil, which is a rich nutrient made from the milk of cows grazing on rapidly growing springtime grass.

Cod-Liver Oil (CLO): In the past, European children were given cod-liver oil because it is a good source of Vitamins A, D, K, E and DHA, all of which are important for strong bones, growth, fertility, skin, and brain development. Also available is a high-vitamin fermented cod-liver oil (FCLO), which is made using a process that retains its natural vitamins. According to Dr. Price, the effects of FCLO are enhanced when combined with butter. It is especially important for women and men before conceiving, for women during pregnancy and lactation, and for children. The suggested daily serving of FCLO for pregnant and nursing women is 2 teaspoons CLO providing 20,000 IU vitamin A and 2,000 IU vitamin D per day (mix with water or a beverage).

Organic Fruits and Vegetables: Eat a variety of fruits and vegetables preferably organic, grown locally and in season.

Soaked Grains: By soaking grains for 12 to 24 hours, they become more easily digested. Nowadays many people are sensitive to grains which can cause digestive disturbances and wheat allergies. Soaking breaks down phytic acid, which would otherwise block absorption of minerals in the gut leading to deficiencies and bone loss. Instead of breads with white flour, choose organic whole grains, including sprouted grains such as sprouted wheat tortillas, sourdough rye, steel-cut oats, and organic Wheatena.

Raw Milk and Dairy Products: Milk drinkers should consider consuming raw whole fat milk during pregnancy and lactation. When produced by reputable companies who have healthy cows, raw milk is considered safe and contains many nutritious components that are not found in the standard market variety. Pasteurization destroys valuable enzymes and nutrients, changing the quality of the milk which can trigger an immune response that leads to milk intolerance and increases health problems for the mother, such as allergies, asthma, and frequent upper respiratory infections.

Bone Broth (also known as chicken soup): Stock made from the bones of chicken, meat, and fish are nutritious. Use the broth as a base for stews and soups, or sip on its own. Old-fashioned chicken soup has been used as a cure-all for colds, flu, and a myriad of health problems. Gelatin-rich broths also aid digestion, and are important for those with intestinal disorders and many chronic illnesses.

Fermented Foods: In the past, foods were fermented as a way to preserve them for longer periods. Known as lacto-fermentation, lactic acid is produced through the fermentation process and works by inhibiting bacteria from spoiling the food. Advantages of consuming fermented foods include easier digestion of vegetables and increased vitamins and enzymes known to have antibiotic and anti-cancer properties. In addition, it helps support the healthy bacteria in the intestine (similar to probiotics). Fermented foods such as sauerkraut to kimchi are easy to make at home. Cultured milks including yogurt, kefir, and sour cream are also healthy options.

Organic Meats, Poultry, Fish, Eggs, and Organ Meats: Consider the sources when you purchase meats, poultry, fish, and eggs. Wild fish, free-range chicken, grass-fed beef, and eggs without antibiotics or growth hormones are a priority and can be consumed in moderate amounts. Although no longer a staple in the American kitchen, organ meats such as liver, kidney, and heart have been valued for being rich in vitamins, fatty acids, and minerals. The suggested serving is 2 to 4 ounces fresh liver (beef, lamb, chicken, duck, turkey, goose) preferably from pasture-raised animals, once or twice per week.

Healthy Fats: Not all fats are created equal, and fats from animals and vegetable sources are important for energy supply, cell membranes, and the production of hormones in the body. All fats should be whole, full fat; avoid consuming low-fat or nonfat products. For cooking, use butter, lard (pigs), chicken fat, palm oil, palm kernel oil, and coconut oil (olive oil is also okay at low temperatures). Use olive oil, expeller pressed flax oil (in small amounts), expeller pressed sesame oil, and peanut oils (in small amounts) for salads and steamed vegetables. Junk food and processed food contains hydrogenated oils (partially hydrogenated, also known as trans fats) which are linked to cancer, heart disease, sterility, learning disabilities, osteoporosis, and growth problems. Avoid soy, corn, safflower, cottonseed, grape seed, and canola oils.

Avoid Processed Foods, Cereals, Crackers, and Soy: Eat whole foods. Avoid white refined foods (flours, rice, and sugar), cereals and crackers (including organic brands, goldfish crackers, and rice cakes), artificial sweeteners, and soy products. Cereals are made using an extrusion process of high temperature and intense pressure which destroys nutrients, causes oils to go rancid, and makes the food difficult to digest. White flour is broken down into the body like sugar, and contributes to moodiness and increased cravings. Most soy is manufactured in a way that alters proteins and increases levels of carcinogens. Soy can also lead to deficiencies of vitamin D and calcium, and hypothyroidism, and soy-based formula has the estrogenic equivalent of five birth control pills per day.

Sugar and Salt: Read the labels. Avoid the use of refined white sugar and artificial sweeteners. For baking, use rapadura (raw cane sugar), pure maple syrup, raw honey, or molasses. Stevia is a sweetener made from the leaves of the Stevia rebaudiana plant. It is sweeter than sugar and can be used in beverages, appetizers, and desserts. Because natural sweeteners such as honey and maple syrup can affect blood sugar and contribute to sweet cravings, use them in moderation two to three times per week as part of a meal. Use unrefined salt (i.e. Celtic sea salt, Himalayan crystal salt). Standard iodized table salt lacks important minerals due to manufacturing, and contains additives (including sugar).

Glycemic Index

Eating healthy also consists of consuming foods that have an optimal glycemic index (GI), which is a ranking of carbohydrates in food. The lower GI foods are recommended during pregnancy because they are digested slower, thereby producing a more gradual rise in blood sugar and improved insulin levels. Lower GI foods include carrots, peanuts, apples, grapefruit, peas, and lentils. Higher GI foods include white rice, white bread, white baked potato, and brown rice.

Pesticides and Food

Pesticides and insecticides are meant to exterminate insects by attacking their nervous system. For this reason it is especially important to avoid consuming foods treated with pesticides and avoid exposure to household pesticides in the first trimester of pregnancy when your baby's nervous system is developing. The *American Journal of Public Health,* as well as other medical journals, has acknowledged the link between pesticides and birth defects, as well as complications in pregnancy including miscarriage.

Below are a few tips for reducing your family's exposure to pesticides on produce:
- ❀ Wash and peel fruits and vegetables
- ❀ Eat organic when possible, especially when choosing foods with the highest pesticide residues
- ❀ Choose local produce

The Smart Produce Guide (from the Institute for Agriculture and Trade Policy) lists produce with the highest to lowest pesticide residues. Eat organic whenever choosing the following produce, which are highest in pesticides: apples, grapes (imported), nectarine, peaches, pears, red raspberries, strawberries, bell peppers, carrots, celery, green beans, hot peppers, potatoes, and spinach. Additional information can be found online through the Institute for Agriculture and Trade Policy.

The Minnesota Smart Fish Guide offers information about fish, including ones we should avoid because of toxins such as mercury, flame retardants, and other chemicals that can build up in some fish leading to health risks, especially for fetuses and children. These include freshwater bass, carp, catfish, muskie, Northern pike (over 30"), trout (lake and steelhead), walleye (over 20"), king mackerel, orange roughy, shark, red snapper, swordfish, albacore tuna, and tilefish. Additional online resources include the Institute for Agriculture and Trade Policy Food and Health Program Smart Guide.

Rest and Sleep

Although we do not always make sleep a priority in our busy lives, proper amounts of rest and sleep are important for revitalizing the body, mind, and spirit. In our ancestors' days, when religion played a more prominent role in daily activities, the Sabbath day of rest was taken seriously, as it is known that we are more productive and efficient when we take time out for a quiet period. Many women complain of fatigue during the beginning and end of pregnancy. So much happens within our bodies during our pregnancies, so it is important to listen to your body and give yourself the rest it needs. During my first trimester, I was especially sleepy in the afternoon and appreciated my 15-minute nap because it allowed me to function better throughout the rest of the day. I also knew that my body required more rest while a living human being was being formed within.

Rest according to your body's needs, and when possible, try to be in bed by 10 p.m. when there is a rise of melatonin production. The deepest sleep occurs between 10 p.m. and 2 a.m. According to the National Sleep Foundation, we have internal circadian biological clocks which influence times of sleepiness and alertness. As pregnancy progresses, using pillows may also help a woman find a more comfortable sleeping position. Common complaints that disturb sleep during pregnancy include restless legs, sleep apnea, heartburn (GERD), and frequent urination.

Exercise

We all know the importance of exercise. However, especially during pregnancy the benefits of regular exercise include lowering the risk of high blood pressure and diabetes, preventing excessive weight gain, and shortening labor. Exercise is also known to relieve back ache, bloating, constipation, and swelling. Additionally, a Canadian study found evidence that suggests exercise enhances a baby's brain development. In a group of pregnant women who exercised for 20 minutes three times per week, researchers measured the brain activity of the newborns in the exercise group, which showed more mature brain activity corresponding to that of babies of 6 to 8 months of age.

Being pregnant, giving birth, and caretaking our children require energy and stamina. If you are not accustomed to some form of activity, begin now. Start slowly and work your way up, from cleaning the house and walking the dog to taking an exercise class. Whatever you do, it is important to participate in physical activity that is enjoyable, and hopefully can be continued after your baby arrives. During my pregnancy, I enjoyed prenatal yoga, as it was the one place I could exercise with other expectant mommies. In addition to getting exercise, I made lasting friendships at my prenatal yoga class and learned a lot of tips about pregnancy and birth—many of which I share with others to this day. Walking is an excellent exercise especially during pregnancy. It is good for endurance and relieves stiffness, and a brisk walk keeps the blood flowing. During my prenatal yoga class, our teacher Gurmukh, reminded us, "Walk, walk, and walk some more!"

Pelvic Tilt

A common exercise taught in prenatal yoga classes is the pelvic tilt, also known as the cat-cow stretch. This movement is especially important in the second and third trimester. According to Yoga guru Kristin McGee, the pelvic tilt "opens the back [and] relieves tension in [the] hips, shoulders, and lower back. It also helps build core strength and pelvic floor stability." Although this pose benefits everyone, during pregnancy it helps promote circulation and encourages the baby to stay in an optimal position or to move into the best one for labor. The optimal fetal position is the occipital anterior position in which the head is down, facing mother's back, chin is tucked, and her back lies along mother's belly. In this position, she has greater ease fitting through the pelvis. As with any new exercise, it is always advisable to check with your healthcare provider before beginning.

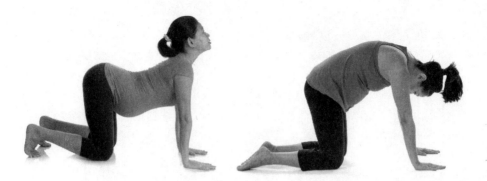

How to do a Pelvic Tilt

Begin on hands and knees in a tabletop position on the floor. Inhale; arch the back, lifting the sitting bones toward the ceiling. Exhale, tucking the tail bone, and straighten the back to neutral position. Repeat 40 cycles slowly on a daily basis (can be done in sets of 10 to 20 throughout the day).

Your Relationships and Stress

Our relationships with others, and especially with our spouse or partner, profoundly influence our lives. Before your baby is born, it is ideal to spend quality time with your partner because during the first few months (at least), everyone's focus will be on the baby and your relationships can become secondary.

During pregnancy, hormonal changes and general discomfort and fatigue can heighten mood changes and add extra stress when relating to others. Stress can lead to health problems, and in pregnancy can cause a woman to deliver prematurely (before 37 weeks). Premature birth can lead to complications such as developmental delays, learning disorders, and chronic lung conditions. In addition, stress in utero may increase the propensity for your baby to develop health conditions in adulthood such as high blood pressure, heart disease, and diabetes. Just as it is important to honor the physical and emotional changes that occur during pregnancy, so it is also important to ask for help, support, and guidance when the stress becomes overwhelming. (See Chapter 4 for more guidance.)

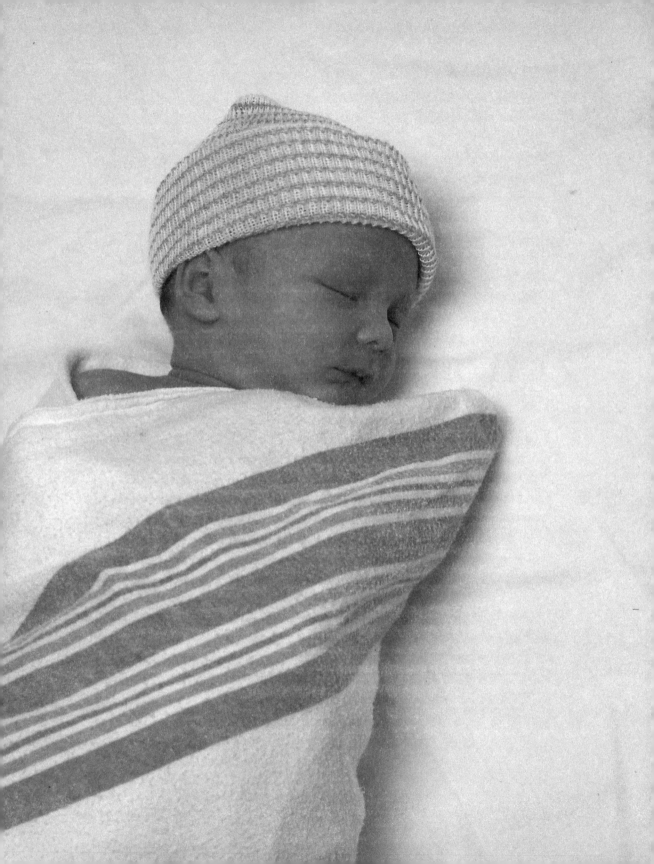

Making Decisions: Practitioner, Birthplace, and Prenatal Tests

Midwives to Medical Doctors: Different Models of Care

FROM THE DOCTOR'S DESK

Just a few days before her due date, Livia began to sense that her obstetrician was not the right practitioner for her. The doctor had been monitoring her for the past week because of minor fetal heart-rate changes. She felt at odds with him, as he was pushing her to have a C-section which she intuitively felt was not justified. After consulting with me about her apprehension with the way things were progressing, I encouraged her to seek a second opinion. Three days later she had a beautiful natural birth in the hospital with her new obstetrician.

Stories like this are not uncommon in my practice. With changes in sophisticated communication systems and the Internet, patients are savvier and more knowledgeable compared to earlier generations who never questioned doctors. Patients are interested in partnering with their practitioner for their healthcare, and actively seek out a patient-practitioner relationship in which they can freely engage in discussions and ask questions at ease. Sometimes, people choose a practitioner who meets their needs, then with time realize those needs have changed, and move on to other doctors. Sometimes, as in Livia's case, it happens at the 11th hour. People investigate many things in life from food ingredients to mobile phone companies, and so it should be with your healthcare providers.

Increasingly, expectant parents are turning to mother-friendly practitioners (and institutions) for individualized attention and respect for the natural birth process. But whether you are inclined to choose a midwife or doctor, the patient-practitioner relationship ideally marks the beginning of a trusted relationship. For some families, financial concerns help dictate choice of practitioner and venue. With insurance companies taking a greater role in determining available doctors and midwives, many families find they are "shopping" for a practitioner in ways their parents' and grandparents' generations never did.

The concept of midwifery was totally foreign to my upbringing and my medical training. Yet, after I had done my research, I knew that I wanted to deliver at home with a midwife. I decided early in my first pregnancy that I wanted to enjoy my experience, and not try to orchestrate it. So I decided to sit back, be a pregnant woman, and place my care with a thoughtfully chosen team, from my birth instructor and midwife to my backup doctor. In a midwife, I was looking for a more holistic approach with someone who viewed me as an individual. I appreciated the time she spent with me during visits, and her patience during my labor.

The Midwife Approach

Midwifery is an optimal model of care for most births. As the majority of births are normal, midwives are experts trained in normal birth. The role of the midwife is to provide prenatal care throughout pregnancy, deliver babies, and assist in the postpartum period. Midwives are well trained to deal with complications when they arise; however, they defer high-risk cases and complications to medical doctors, specifically obstetricians.

According to the Mother-Friendly Childbirth Initiative, "Midwives attend the vast majority of births in those industrialized countries with the best perinatal outcomes, yet in the United States, midwives are the principal attendants at only a small percentage of births." In other countries, most women never see an obstetrician unless a complication arises. With modern medicine, the role of the midwife as primary caretaker for pregnant women was eclipsed by obstetricians, especially in the United States. However, the presence of midwives throughout American hospitals is now becoming more commonplace.

There are various training paths for midwives. *Certified nurse midwives* (CNM) are registered nurses with midwifery accreditation, and can also act as primary healthcare providers for women from adolescence through menopause. They can perform physical exams, prescribe medications, and order laboratory tests. Although they can deliver in any venue, most hospital-based midwives are CNM trained. In addition to CNMs, the *licensed direct-entry midwife* (LDM) is trained in midwifery only, and no prior credentials are needed. They specialize in home birth and at work at birth centers in the United States; however, in many western European countries, they attend the majority of normal hospital births. LDMs can be graduates of accredited education programs or are trained through apprenticeships.

The midwifery model of care encompasses the very definition of natural childbirth, as it is in accordance with the way in which Mother Nature intended for women to give birth. Compared to medical doctors, there are inherent differences in the way in which midwives are trained and the method of practice. In general, midwives spend more time with a laboring woman than do doctors, who often rely on hospital nurses (or in-house midwives) for the majority of time a woman is in labor, and usually arrive only for delivery. Becoming more prevalent in the United States are the hospital-based midwives. For many pregnant women, having a midwife deliver in the hospital offers the "best of both worlds." In the hospital setting, similar to obstetricians, midwife-assisted deliveries have the capability to order pain medications, including epidurals. According to midwife Ina May Gaskin, "Good research shows that when the midwifery model of care is applied, between eighty-five and ninety-five percent of healthy women will safely give birth without surgery or instruments such as forceps and vacuum-extractors."

Most importantly, the midwifery model of care is about being *with the woman*, supporting her during the contractions, and assisting her with different positions and techniques that help manage the discomfort. Being familiar with the varying pace of a woman's labor, midwives are patient and acknowledge the importance of an undisturbed birth. In the postpartum period, they often assist mother and baby with continuity of care including breastfeeding. The midwife's expertise (along with simple acts and gestures) adds up, and can help avoid or reduce the need for medications for induction or pain. In fact, research shows that midwife-assisted births carry fewer rates of interventions such as episiotomy, epidurals, fetal monitoring, and cesarean section. While I am a big fan of midwives, it should be noted that there are also excellent physicians who provide personalized care and support a woman's decision for a natural birth. Although rare, there are even some M.D.s who offer home and birth center deliveries. (At a doula meeting, the panel referred to M.D.s who perform natural birth as "Midwives in Disguise"!)

Home Birth

Without having the specific words to describe it, I yearned to give birth naturally, at home. The home environment is one that encourages natural birth: freedom to move, eat, drink, sleep, and bathe. Without being pressured, I did not have to contend with traffic, hospital staff, or unfamiliar sights, smells, and sounds. Frankly, when one plans a home birth, one is committing to a labor and delivery that is natural; free of medications and most interventions commonly found in the hospital. At the same time, I was confident with my midwife's training and expertise. Beforehand, my midwife gave us a list of birth kit supplies to have on hand. Depending upon your midwife, prenatal care is either done at an office, or in your home. During home birth, the midwife is accompanied by an assistant and will come prepared with birth equipment and medical supplies including oxygen in the event of an emergency.

In the United States, mention the word "home birth" and you are apt to receive more than a few charged responses from people ignorant of the home birth process. However, outside the U.S. it is more commonly accepted and is even well integrated into the healthcare system. Home birth remains controversial among such medical organizations as the American Congress of Obstetricians and Gynecologists (ACOG). According to a large study from the *British Medical Journal*, the outcomes for planned low-risk home births were associated with lower rates of medical intervention compared to those in the hospital. In addition, childbirth and newborn mortality rates were similarly low in both home and hospital births. The researchers concurred there was a high degree of safety and maternal satisfaction reported with home birth. A cost analysis found that in the United States uncomplicated vaginal hospital births cost three times more than an uncomplicated home birth with a midwife. Their conclusion, "Our study of certified professional midwives suggests that they achieve good outcomes among low-risk women without routine use of expensive hospital intervention."

For many women, the choice to have a home birth is based on the fact that it is *at home*: the same place where baby was conceived, baby is delivered. Compared to a hospital, many women prefer the home environment because it is familiar and comfortable, there is no risk of infection from sick people, nor are there limitations of visiting hours for family and friends. The cons of home birth include the possibility of incurring more out-of-pocket expenses due to lower reimbursement from your insurance company. Home birth carries the lowest intervention rate, so another downside for some women is that there is no epidural or standard pain medication given because these medications can increase risk to baby and mother. Sometimes, women are transported to the hospital during labor. There can be many reasons for this, but usually this is done if labor is not progressing, and on rare occasions, because of an emergency. Most of the time, women transferred to the hospital are accompanied by the midwife for support and advocacy.

Birth Centers

Birth centers are usually independent and privately owned; staffed with midwives, they offer a home-like environment. They can also include birthing tubs and showers for laboring mothers. Birth centers are a wonderful alternative to a home birth, when the home may not appropriate due to size or lack of privacy. Some birth centers are connected to a hospital and offer expectant couples the choice to birth in a homey environment, often with birth tubs. Midwives affiliated with a birth center connected to a hospital may still be obligated to follow routine hospital policies, although rates of intervention are usually lower (see "Interventions" in Chapter 3).

The Doctor Approach

As the daughter of a medical doctor, I grew up believing that when I was pregnant I would have an obstetrician and deliver in the hospital. At the time, I did not realize there were choices. One benefit of working with physicians is that they are well trained in dealing with high-risk medical problems, whether they are from pre-existing maternal conditions like epilepsy or heart disease, or from pregnancy-related complications such as preeclampsia. Obstetrics is a surgical specialty, and obstetricians receive training in oncology, urology, pelvic reconstruction, infertility, family planning, and maternal fetal medicine. Many doctors are unfamiliar with the concept of a natural, undisturbed birth, and believe that labor usually requires medication. I heard a doctor once complain that being with a laboring woman was "boring." Being with a woman in labor requires patience, because in many ways there may not be much for the practitioner to do. Midwife Ina May Gaskin commented, vaginal deliveries in a hospital setting would be better understood by obstetricians if "they would be able to connect birthing to the animal world and not make birthing a procedure."

Many American women prefer working with an obstetrician based on comfort level and familiarity. However, what many people do not realize is that the doctor often arrives in time for delivery of the baby, which is at the end of labor. With rising healthcare costs and lower insurance reimbursements, medical doctors are seeing more patients but spending less time with each one. Similarly, labor and delivery nurses are assigned to specific patients, and come in to check at regular intervals, but they are busy juggling several patients simultaneously. Ironically, a woman may spend a significant amount of time laboring alone in the hospital room without much support. For this reason, it is important to consider having a birth team which may include your partner, a family member, and/or a doula.

Hospital Setting

As with any form of medical care, there are pros and cons to giving birth in a hospital setting. In the U.S., there are both private and public hospital institutions, and their use is dependent on insurance coverage and financial needs. In a private setting, the benefits can include nicer accommodations, your choice of obstetrician, and a private room with overnight stay for your partner. Hospital-based midwives are usually more apt to follow the standard obstetrical model. Fortunately, a few private hospitals are beginning to offer more private midwifery privileges. On the downside, there may be more out-of-pocket expenses because the medical model in a private institution leads to the highest rate of intervention, including cesarean section. The public hospital setting is less expensive with fewer interventions; however it has higher neonatal intensive care unit (NICU) transfers for premature and sick babies. Still, some public hospitals offer excellent midwifery programs for labor and delivery care. In general, hospitals are a place for sick people who seek diagnosis, treatment, or care; and some laboring women are offended when they enter the hospital in labor and are immediately placed in a wheelchair and treated as if sick.

I have great respect for the state of pregnancy, and especially childbirth. I have been honored to be present at most of my friends' deliveries, and have witnessed wonderful births at both home or in the hospital. The choice of birthplace is personal, and is based on one's desires, as well as need.

Find Your Comfort Zone

Whether you deliver at home, at a birth center, or in a hospital, it is important to find *your* comfort zone. In making these decisions, you will hear other people's well-meaning opinions, whether they are asked or not. But ultimately it should be a place where you can feel most relaxed and secure, in order to be able to surrender to this incredible life-giving experience.

Doulas

Having support during one of the most momentous experiences of your life is vital. In the past, women were surrounded by other women—a midwife, mother, and women of the village. Nowadays, fathers are playing a more active role in the birth experience and, along with family and friends, can offer great support during childbirth and the postpartum period. However, many eager friends and family members may not have the experience or sensitivity to deal with the birth process. At my first birth, my mother had never witnessed another woman's birth before. Although she was supportive, she was not able to give me much guidance.

Fortunately for mothers-to-be, professionals are available to offer support during birth and afterwards. If you are planning to deliver in the hospital and want a natural birth, then bring a good support team. Today, more parents in my office practice work with doulas who are trained to support a mother during labor, as well as during the first days and weeks following. *Doula* is a Greek word that refers to the main female servant in a household. According to Dr. Marshall Klaus, author of *Mothering the Mother,* the evidence shows that women who labor with a doula at their side have lower rates of cesarean sections (50%), and forceps use (40%), and there are fewer requests for epidurals (60%), and shorter labors (25%). Doulas are trained in the birth process and postpartum period. Although they do not actually deliver babies, their nurturing presence can enable a woman to smoothly transition into motherhood. Doulas stay by the woman to make her experience more comfortable, whether through massage, reassurance, physical comfort measures, or even assisting the father-to-be or other family members. Especially helpful for hospital births, doulas are familiar with the hospital setting and can advocate for the mother and family; this is a great boon in dealing with the nursing staff (as well as the doctor).

If having a natural birth is an integral part of your birth plan and you are delivering in a hospital setting, strongly consider hiring a doula as part of your birth team. If you are planning on delivering with a midwife, a doula may not be needed as the midwife typically has time to support the laboring woman and is usually sufficient. No matter what you decide, it is best to discuss this with your practitioner ahead of time, and trust your instinct!

Choosing a Practitioner

It is important to know your practitioner's philosophy, as his or her ideology can greatly affect the outcome of your birth. Many women choose a practitioner based on friend's recommendations, but the ideal practitioner for your friend may or may not be right for you. Some people stay with a doctor they have been seeing as a gynecologist. In general, if sometime during the pregnancy unforeseen events arise that negatively impact your relationship with the practitioner, it is appropriate to get a second opinion or change to another provider. Many practitioners offer monthly introductory meetings, and it is worth your while to interview several of them. In addition to expertise, it is important to take into account your personal observations and instincts about bedside manner, nursing, and support staff. Whether you are looking for a midwife or a doctor, make a list of questions that are important to you.

Consider asking the following questions, especially if you are interested in a natural birth:

* What is your birth philosophy?
* What are your thoughts about going beyond the due date?
* What are your thoughts about doula support?
* Questions about interventions:
    * What percentage of your clients delivers without medication?
    * What is your rate of epidurals?
    * What is your rate of episiotomy?
    * How do you feel about eating and drinking during labor?
    * Are IVs used routinely, or only if medically needed?
    * Do you allow intermittent monitoring once I'm in labor at the hospital? (i.e., 20 minutes on and 40 minutes off)
    * Once my water breaks, how do you handle time limits before going to the hospital?
    * What is your C-section rate?
    * What are your thoughts about cord clamping?
* What is your rate of transfer to a hospital? (For both home and birth centers.)
* What are your fees?
* Do you accept insurance?

Informed Choice: Making Decisions Using Your B.R.A.I.N.

In the United States we pride ourselves on the ability to offer women the most sophisticated obstetrical healthcare in a state-of-the-art environment. At various stages of pregnancy, different testing is done—some tests are routine while others are elective—but the important thing to note is that *you* have a choice about which tests to undergo. Many women do not know much about the tests or procedures that are available and instead rely on their practitioners, assuming that any information one receives is beneficial and harmless. As a result, many women have undergone testing without fully considering all the implications.

The American Congress of Obstetricians and Gynecologists (ACOG) recommends that practitioners provide patients with information about tests and procedures so that they can make an informed decision. However, practitioners often assume patients understand all the details about the tests and unfortunately do not always share the necessary information. Many childbirth educators, including the International Childbirth Education Association, adopt the BRAIN acronym (benefits, risks, alternative, intuition, nothing) in making a decision. Taking time to consider your options can offer clarity in all aspects of life, especially during pregnancy, birth, and beyond.

On ethical grounds, patients are supposed to be given information in a format that is easily understood and done without obligation. Yet, sometimes the information can be confusing and conflicting, and is dependent upon the healthcare providers' point of view. Practitioners give advice based on expertise as well as their subjective experiences in life. Our generation is savvy, we have access to information on the Internet, which is sometimes a blessing and sometimes not. We are different from our parents who never questioned the medical profession. I encourage you to partner with your practitioners. If you do not know or understand, ask questions. Before undergoing any blood test, screen, or procedure use the BRAIN acronym and ask the following questions (as well as any others you may have):

- ❀ Benefits: What are the benefits to my baby and me?
  - ❀ Do I understand what the test or screening is for?
  - ❀ Is it necessary, routine, or elective?
  - ❀ How will this help my pregnancy or labor?
- ❀ Risks: What are the risks to my baby and me?
  - ❀ How will this affect us?
  - ❀ If the test result is unfavorable, what are the implications and choices?
- ❀ Alternatives: Have I been informed about similar or alternative tests?
  - ❀ Do I have another choice?
- ❀ Intuition/Instinct: What is my gut feeling?
  - ❀ Does the information make sense?
- ❀ Nothing/Need Time/Not Now: What if I decide to do nothing and wait?
  - ❀ Can I wait on this decision (to allow time to discuss this with my family and think it through)?

Remember, this is *your* pregnancy and *your* baby, and your informed choice is the most important—even if you are not in the medical field!

Prenatal Tests: What to Do with the Information

We live in a time where we have much information at our fingertips, but in some cases it can feel like information overload. Additionally, expectant couples often complain about a lack of guidance on what to expect from various prenatal tests and which tests are truly necessary—in other words, many patients are not well informed when they consent to prenatal testing. After announcing my pregnancy with joy, my parents encouraged me to undergo prenatal tests such as an ultrasound and amniocentesis so that I could know as much as possible about my baby, even if the results were deleterious. Although they knew my husband and I would not consider termination, my parents believed it would be helpful for us to know about any complications ahead of time, so that we could be prepared. Ultimately, we decided that we wanted to enjoy the pregnancy, without any undue worry, and if anything needed to be done at birth, we would address it at that time. On this note, I understood the Mayo Clinic's opening comment about prenatal testing, "Pregnancy is a time of great anticipation—and anxiety."

In recent years, the medical model of prenatal care has made great strides in technology, and as a result there are many prenatal tests performed during pregnancy. From screening tests such as ultrasound and blood tests to diagnostic procedures like amniocentesis, these tests provide information to practitioners about the development and growth of the baby. Expectant couples look forward to the tests as they appreciate receiving information about their baby's progress. Although everyone expects to hear good news, many are unprepared to receive a negative result. Doctors routinely order tests based on current recommendations throughout pregnancy, often assuming that the tests are advantageous and that couples would terminate following a poor diagnosis. Most pregnant women do not realize that many prenatal tests are elective, not routine. Many consent to the tests without fully knowing the implications, as it was not explained to them. Furthermore, prenatal testing is quite sophisticated and provides both practitioner and patient with a plethora of information, some of which are incidental findings without any symptoms, but still can lead to a great deal of anxiety.

Before consenting to any screening and diagnostic tests, it is advisable to consider the consequences. Faced with an abnormal diagnosis from prenatal testing, some couples are prepared to continue with pregnancy, while others would terminate, and still other couples do not know how they would respond. Knowing in advance what you would with the information from the prenatal tests is important, because this will help guide you, and allow you to choose which tests are necessary or unnecessary. In my case, we knew ahead of time that we would not consider a termination, and for this reason, many of the prenatal tests which were offered were obsolete in my mind.

Prenatal tests include both screening and diagnostic tests. Screening tests are more general and predict the likelihood for a potential condition. If a screening test is positive or there are factors that indicate possible high risk due to age or a pre-existing medical condition, then a diagnostic test can be done which is more definitive.

Ultrasound

Ultrasound is used to view the fetus during pregnancy. It began in the 1800s as a sonar device used to measure distance under water with sound waves. In World War I, it was used for submarine navigation. In addition to its imaging capability, ultrasound became known for its heating qualities and destructive effects on animal tissues in the laboratory. In medicine, ultrasound began to be used in the 1940s by physical therapists for applications such as increasing local blood flow and reducing inflammation. By the 1960s, ultrasound began its use as an imaging device which replaced x-rays for fetal imaging. Prior to this, abdominal x-rays were used in pregnancy to determine the baby's position, until Dr. Alice Stewart warned that the low-dose radiation increased the rate of childhood cancer. Initially, ultrasound began as a way to screen and diagnose high-risk conditions; however, it is now used routinely in most pregnancies.

Ultrasound in pregnancy works by emitting ultra-high frequency sound waves, beyond the range of human hearing, which create an image of the fetus in the womb. From a transducer (or a probe) placed within the vagina in early pregnancy or on the surface of the abdomen thereafter, sound waves are emitted at millions of cycles per second. (Modern ultrasound energy intensities are higher now than in earlier decades.) Ultrasounds are used at various stages of pregnancy to assess both mother and baby.

The following are the different types of ultrasound:

Transvaginal Scan: Done in early pregnancy, before 8 weeks. Considered to be high exposure levels of ultrasound due to close proximity of the probe to the early developing fetus. Some women complain that the wand placed in the vagina can be uncomfortable, invasive, or embarrassing.

Standard Scan: Traditional abdominal ultrasound, which generates 2-D images of the developing fetus. Used after 8 weeks of pregnancy.

Doppler Ultrasound (Doptone): Handheld device on the abdomen used by many obstetricians and midwives. Used to monitor baby's heart beat and to study blood flow through the umbilical cord. In addition, there are waterproof Dopplers which can be used in a water birth to monitor baby's heart rate.

Electronic Fetal Monitor: (See Chapter 3.) Used in late pregnancy and during labor to monitor the baby and her or his heartbeat. Often used for hours continuously, and considered to be high-exposure level.

3-D Ultrasound/4-D Transabdominal Ultrasound: The 3-D ultrasound generates three-dimensional images of the developing fetus, around the 19th–20th week of pregnancy. A 4D ultrasound is similar to 3-D, but it creates a live video or movie in which one can see the baby's body and facial movements. Both are used for high-risk pregnancy, although they are growing in popularity, and are even found in some shopping malls!

Benefits of Ultrasound

Ultrasound uses are twofold. Prenatal ultrasound is commonly used routinely, such as in confirming pregnancy early on or inspecting fetal organs and development at approximately 18 to 20 weeks. Ultrasounds are also used to gain information on specific conditions such as bleeding, growth concerns, or the baby's position in late pregnancy. In addition, many expectant parents look forward with great anticipation to "see" their baby on ultrasound.

In general, ultrasounds are performed for the following reasons:
- ❀ Assess uterus, ovaries, placenta
- ❀ Confirm pregnancy
- ❀ Detect multiple births
- ❀ Calculate due date
- ❀ Inspect fetal organs for growth and development
- ❀ Check gender
- ❀ Verify fetal position and breech presentation
- ❀ Inspect the placenta and placement
- ❀ Evaluate levels of amniotic fluids
- ❀ Identify pelvic abnormalities of the mother
- ❀ "See" the baby

Risks of Ultrasound

As sound waves are used instead of radiation, doctors consider ultrasound to be safe and noninvasive. For this reason, risks are often not discussed, nor considered. However, according to the American Pregnancy Association, "The long term effects of repeated ultrasound exposures on the fetus are not fully known. It is recommended that ultrasound only be used if medically indicated." A study with 15,000 low-risk pregnancies concluded the use of routine ultrasound is debatable and does not improve outcome and therefore should be done selectively. These warnings are clearly not heeded, as it is estimated that most women in the United States will have a routine ultrasound sometime during pregnancy, and often multiple times. Moreover, ultrasound is becoming more commonplace, as women in 2006 were twice as likely to have an ultrasound in pregnancy compared to 1995. In addition, commercial ultrasound services have surfaced as a place where expectant families can make appointments for various packages from heartbeat check and gender peeks, to deluxe packages with 30-minute 3D and 4D sessions.

False Positives

One of the risks of having an ultrasound, is receiving information about the results of the scan, without knowing how to decipher them. Routine ultrasound is not able to detect all abnormalities, and there can be errors in predicting a baby's gender. According to Dr. Sarah Buckley, one study showed that routine ultrasound detects between 17 percent and 80 percent of major abnormalities, and another study from Brisbane missed approximately 40 percent of them. In addition, women have been given information about abnormalities, when in fact the baby was fine; these are known as "false positive" findings. In some cases, false positive findings have resulted in the abortion of normal babies. Needless to say, receiving an abnormal result is a great source of anxiety and stress for parents, another example of the nocebo effect.

The Heating Effects of Ultrasound

Studies have shown that women exposed to heat, such as from hot tubs or saunas, in early pregnancy have a greater risk of birth defects. However, it is recognized that ultrasound also can cause heating. During ultrasound, some of the waves are reflected while others are absorbed. The reflected waves generate the image, but the absorbed waves generate heat, causing thermal changes in the tissue and resulting in gas bubbles. This can lead to small local gas pockets in affected tissues which collapse, leaving cavities, known as *cavitation*. According to the National Council on Radiation Protection and Measurements (NCRPM), some machines cause temperatures to rise if the probe is left in one spot, rather than continuously moved, which may prevent harmful elevations in temperature. Theoretically, high temperature from ultrasound use can lead to production of reactive chemicals such as free radicals, which could potentially cause genetic and cell damage. The committee recommends that ultrasound technicians be aware of these risks and avoid leaving a probe in one focal area for a prolonged period of time (more than 10 minutes).

Determining the exact risks of ultrasound is complicated by the fact that ethically, scientific research and experiments cannot be conducted on pregnant women. According to researchers from Yale University, exposure to ultrasound waves disrupts brain development in fetal mice. Although the ultrasound wave levels used in the experiment were beyond those used by obstetricians, the authors said it should raise concerns about use of commercial "keepsake" ultrasound services. Although there is no evidence that it could affect brain development in human babies, "the findings indicate a need for further study and caution with nonmedical exposure."

Considerations

While doctors receive a plethora of data from scans, the expectant parents are given results which can be confusing and anxiety provoking. Most physicians assume that detection of severe fetal abnormalities will be cause for termination. Because this is rarely discussed ahead of time, many couples remain uninformed about and unprepared to deal with the implications of ultrasound findings. For example a relatively common finding in the 2nd trimester ultrasound scan is enlargement in part of the kidney (known as fetal pyelactasis), found more commonly in males and also considered a soft sign for chromosomal abnormalities.

Although the vast majority (96%) of cases are benign and resolve spontaneously in the first year of life, findings like these are an enormous cause of stress and anxiety for the family, and for no reason. For women who would not consider a termination, the information from a routine ultrasound is unnecessary. According to Beverley Beech, the chairman of the Association for Improvements in Maternity Services, "I am not sure at all that the benefits of ultrasound scans outweigh the downsides. We should be advising women to think very, very carefully before they have scans at all." Most expectant couples are excited to be able to "see" their baby, not realizing that one of the purposes of the scan is to look for abnormalities. After receiving this information, "Women can feel pressured to have a termination, or at the least feel some emotional distancing from their "abnormal" baby," writes Dr. Sarah Buckley. Research about ultrasound has been inconclusive, but has also suggested the following adverse effects:

- ❀ Increased left-handedness in children (according to researchers, exposure to ultrasound in utero increases the risk of left-handedness in males, which suggests that ultrasound affects the fetal brain)
- ❀ Cell abnormalities
- ❀ Damage to myelin sheath covering the nerves
- ❀ Early labor

❀ Low birth weight
❀ Restricted fetal growth
❀ Premature birth
❀ Miscarriage
❀ Poorer health in newborns, and perinatal death
❀ Increased learning disabilities
❀ Delayed speech
❀ Epilepsy

It is presumed that use of ultrasound and the information it provides is considered valuable and essential for every pregnancy. As with many of the tests and procedures performed during pregnancy, it is important to consider the risks, benefits, and implications of the test. Ultrasound is an elective test, it is *not* mandatory. During my pregnancies, I declined all ultrasound and Doppler tests, deferring instead to the archaic obstetric stethoscope which meant my midwife could hear my baby's heartbeat by my 20th week, late compared to ultrasound standards!

Even my parents tried to convince me to have an ultrasound, as they considered their grandchild-to-be worthy of state-of-the-art ultrasound technology. As I told them, I made my decision based on several factors. Many people were given too much medical information that did not necessarily improve pregnancy outcome and only caused anguish for the family. I chose to trust my body's internal wisdom, rather than rely on a routine ultrasound. My colleagues reassured me that ultrasound was harmless. However, I knew there had been many instances in the past decades in which pregnant women were reassured by their doctors that use of x-ray, DES (diethylstilbestrol), and thalidomide were harmless, only to learn after the fact, that there were side effects. (The medication DES is a synthetic estrogen that was prescribed from 1938 to 1971 for pregnant women who had experienced miscarriages and premature deliveries. Although it was considered safe, it was found to be linked to health risks in both sons and daughters including risk of vaginal cancer (in offspring), breast cancer, pregnancy complications, and infertility. The German drug, Thalidomide, prescribed in the late 1950s for anxiety, insomnia, and morning sickness in pregnant women, was found to cause malformation of limbs and other birth defects.) In addition, I knew that I would not consider termination, so I felt the information was unwarranted. Being somewhat old-fashioned, I looked forward to finding out whether my baby was a boy or girl, at birth! And in the end, I just wanted to enjoy my pregnancies.

But let's be realistic. Living in our modern world, most pregnant women will undergo a minimum number of ultrasounds.

If you are having an ultrasound, consider the following:

- ❁ Use ultrasound sparingly and avoid unnecessary scans
- ❁ Work with an experienced ultrasonography technician at a reputable site
- ❁ Use a scan machine that provides the least exposure in the shortest amount of time

AFP: Triple and Quadruple Screening

Benefits of AFP

Alpha-fetoprotein (AFP), also known as the maternal serum AFP (MSAFP), is a protein which is secreted by the fetus' liver and excreted into the mother's bloodstream. It is a blood test that screens for conditions such as defects in the neural tube or abdominal wall, and can also be an indication of Down syndrome. AFP is part of a group of blood tests known as maternal serum triple or quadruple screening which is usually done during the second trimester between 15 and 20 weeks.

The triple screening includes the AFP and the hormones, hCG (human gonadotropin) and unconjugated estriol. This test measures for additional genetic problems such as Down syndrome and neural tube defects.

The quadruple screening is more specific and includes inhibin A hormonal levels, plus the tests of the triple screening. There is also a penta screening, which adds a fifth test called the invasive trophoblast antigen. These multiple blood tests help in identifying the probability that the baby has a chromosomal abnormality such as Down syndrome, trisomy 18, or spina bifida.

Risks of AFP

Screening tests are not specific and require further diagnostic testing, such as amniocentesis, which is recommended for diagnosis if there are positive results. There can also be false-positive results where women with normal babies may experience unnecessary anxiety and worry because of an inaccurate result. Many women over age 35 have received false-positive results because the test is designed to factor in the women's age. Ultimately, many of these women give birth to healthy babies.

Considerations

Although AFP is a simple blood test, it does carry a risk of false positive results which often leads to high anxiety. I would only recommend this test for women who could consider having further testing such as amniocentesis for definitive diagnosis. My husband and I chose not to have this blood test in either of my pregnancies. This included my second pregnancy when I was over 35 years old at the time, which would probably guarantee me an abnormal reading, and I did not want to be burdened with any undue worry because I knew I would not choose any further testing.

Chorionic Villus Sampling (CVS)

Chorionic villus sampling (CVS) is a diagnostic test which checks for certain fetal abnormalities such as Down syndrome, Tay-Sachs disease, cystic fibrosis, and hemophilia. CVS is performed as a biopsy of the chorionic villi found in the mother's placenta. Similar to other tests, it is recommended when there is a family history of genetic disorders or if the mother is 35 years or older. Chorionic villi are found in the placenta, yet also contain the same genetic makeup of the baby. Prior to the procedure, an ultrasound is done to assess the position of both the placenta and the baby. If the placenta is accessible, a thin flexible tube (or catheter) is inserted into the vagina through the cervix and into the placenta for the sampling. Otherwise, the CVS may be performed from the abdomen; this is called a transabdominal CVS. The procedure is usually offered between the 10th and 12th weeks of pregnancy.

Benefits of CVS

In general, CVS is performed for the following reasons:

- ✿ Abnormal ultrasound in the first trimester. If you have an ultrasound early in pregnancy, and there is cause for concern, some women prefer to undergo a CVS to rule out or confirm the ultrasound reading.
- ✿ History of birth defects or genetic disorders. Women who have a family history of birth defects or genetic disorders, or have had a child or a

pregnancy affected by such complications are at higher risk. In addition, a CVS may be performed if the mother or father are known carriers of a genetic disorder.

❧ Women age 35 or older are considered at higher risk for giving birth to children with chromosomal abnormalities, such as Down syndrome.

❧ Earlier results. Some women prefer CVS over amniocentesis because results are available earlier with regard to decision making.

Risks of CVS

❧ Cramping may occur during and after the procedure.

❧ Vaginal bleeding is possible, especially with the transcervical CVS.

❧ Miscarriage risk is one in 100. This risk is increased in the transcervical CVS and if the baby is smaller than average based on gestational age.

❧ Infection may occur from the sampling, which is an invasive procedure.

❧ Because this is an invasive procedure, expectant mothers with Rh negative blood will be given an Rh immunoglobulin shot following the CVS to prevent an Rh sensitization. On occasion during a CVS, baby's blood cells may be released into mother's bloodstream causing antibodies to be produced against the baby.

❧ Research has shown that if the CVS is done too early (i.e., 9th week or earlier) it may increase the chance of defects in baby's limbs (specifically the fingers or toes).

Considerations

Similar to amniocentesis, CVS is an invasive test whose primary aim is detection of genetic conditions and chromosomal abnormalities. I would only recommend this test for women who would consider a termination of pregnancy. There are times when expectant parents may not know how they would respond given the circumstances, and it is important to weigh out the benefits and risks. If you decide to have a CVS, see "Wound Care" in Chapter 5.

Nuchal Translucency Scan (NT)

The nuchal translucency scan, also known as the NT, is a screening ultrasound done between the 11th and 14th weeks of pregnancy. The ultrasound measures the fluid levels at the back of the baby's neck. Babies with increased risk of Down syndrome and other chromosomal conditions, as well as congenital heart conditions, have a tendency to accumulate fluid at the back of the neck during the first trimester. The NT is usually done in conjunction with a blood test known as the first-trimester combined screening. The blood test measures proteins produced by the placenta, free beta-hCG, and PAPP-A (pregnancy associated plasma protein A) both of which are usually higher in babies with Down syndrome.

Benefits of NT
❀ The NT can be performed in the first trimester and is less invasive than other screening and diagnostic tests, such as CVS (chorionic villus sampling) and amniocentesis.
❀ NT screening assesses your baby's risk using a ratio that comes from the results of the ultrasound measurements and blood samples.

Risks of NT
❀ NT is a screening test which gives information on increased risk factors, but it does not provide a definitive diagnosis.
❀ See risks of ultrasound (on page 42).

Considerations
I would recommend this test for women who would consider having further diagnostic tests such as CVS or amniocentesis if the results are abnormal.

Amniocentesis

Amniocentesis is a medical procedure offered to pregnant women during the second trimester for detection of specific types of birth defects and genetic conditions in the fetus. The procedure involves an injection of a local anesthetic followed by the insertion of a needle under ultrasound guidance into the uterus through the belly. A sample of amniotic fluid is taken and sent to the laboratory for analysis.

The test is done during the 15th and 18th week of pregnancy. Amniocentesis is most commonly performed on women who have had an abnormal ultrasound or a family history of genetic conditions or birth defects, and on women who are 35 years or older. Following the procedure, women are prescribed over-the-counter pain medicine to relieve discomfort and cramping. Women are encouraged to rest at home and avoid any strenuous activities, lifting, or sex. Normal activities can be resumed usually a few days thereafter.

Benefits of Amniocentesis

Reasons to consider amniocentesis include detection of Down syndrome, sickle cell disease, cystic fibrosis, muscular dystrophy, Tay-Sachs disease, and other conditions. It is also used to check the baby's gender. Some expectant couples feel reassured by having an amniocentesis.

Risks of Amniocentesis

Amniocentesis is an invasive procedure, yet it is not considered to be high risk. Complications from the procedure are rare but include bleeding, miscarriage (< 1%), clubfoot, preterm labor, and respiratory illnesses in babies at birth, and infection or injury for baby or mother. As with any invasive procedure, the test can be uncomfortable, and it may require more than one needle insertion due to movement of the baby, poor position, or even a Braxton Hicks contraction of the uterus. Following the test, expectant parents are required to wait 2 to 3 weeks for results. For some people, this *waiting game* can be cause for worry (nocebo effect). Although it is not often discussed ahead of time, the medical implication of a serious condition is termination of the baby's life.

Considerations

Amniocentesis provides information about the unborn child including whether the baby may have Down syndrome or a serious fatal condition. Women who receive a positive test are counseled regarding the genetic issues and presented with options, including termination of pregnancy. Although expectant parents may not know how they would respond if they were to receive information of this nature, I encourage you to consider the implications of an amniocentesis beforehand. Because I would not consider terminating my pregnancy, I chose to not have an amniocentesis. An amniocentesis is an elective test, not a routine one, even if you are 35 years or older. In weighing out the risks and benefits of an amniocentesis, women who would not consider termination of pregnancy usually do not have this procedure. If you decide to have an amniocentesis, see "Wound Care" in Chapter 5.

Group Beta Streptococcal Infection (GBS)

Group Beta Streptococcal (GBS) is a bacterium that normally resides in the lower intestine and vagina of 25 percent of healthy women who are considered to be colonized or carriers, usually without symptoms or infection. This is different from the bacteria that causes strep throat, known as Group A Streptococcus. GBS can be passed from a colonized mother to baby during birth, and although rare, can lead to infection which usually occurs within the first seven days of life (known as early onset GBS). GBS is the leading cause of severe infections such as pneumonia, meningitis, and systemic blood infection (sepsis) in newborns. GBS infections affect approximately less than one in two thousand infants yearly in the United States, with a mortality rate of 5 percent in affected infants. The American Congress of Obstetricians and Gynecologists (ACOG) has recommended that all pregnant women be tested for GBS, and women who test positive be given intravenous antibiotics, such as penicillin, every four hours during labor. Nowadays, most practitioners routinely screen for GBS by taking a swab culture from the vagina and rectum during the third trimester from week 35 to 37 when it is most reliable. In a study from the Society of Maternal-Fetal Medicine, researchers showed that the GBS test may not be accurate because some women can have different results between the late trimester screening and a rapid test done at the time of delivery.

There are two types of GBS—early onset (EOGBS), which affects babies up to one week old, and late onset (LOGBS) from one week to 3 months of age. The latter may be due to contact from a colonized person, and is not necessarily linked to a mother's GBS status. EOGBS is the more common of the two. Some practitioners have tried prescribing oral antibiotics to GBS positive women during pregnancy; however, this does not necessarily eliminate the bacteria, and the mother is still given medication during labor.

Risk factors for EOGBS include preterm labor before 37 weeks, premature rupture of the membranes (water breaking), prolonged rupture of membranes (more than 18 hours), fever during labor, bladder infection due to GBS during pregnancy, and women who already have tested positive in previous births or have had a previous baby with GBS.

Benefits of GBS Screening

There are several strategies to GBS screening and preventive treatment. There is debate on whether to prescribe antibiotics routinely for all GBS positive cases (known as the universal approach) or selectively for those with high-risk factors during labor (known as the risk-based approach).

As many of the studies show that the universal approach is more effective, the Centers for Disease Control (CDC) recommends antibiotics for all GBS positive women, whether they are high risk or not. The risk-based approach, which is used outside of the United States (particularly in the United Kingdom) and by many midwives, focuses on treatment of women who have one or more risk factors for GBS. Currently, a rapid-test for GBS during labor is being studied for consideration.

Since the onset of routine screening and preventive treatment of GBS in the mid-1990s, EOGBS has decreased by 80 percent. However, one study found that in spite of universal culturing for GBS and treatment with antibiotics in labor, the researchers were unable to "effect a statistically significant change in the rate of EOGBS sepsis or mortality." Another study found compelling evidence that widespread antibiotic prophylaxis, while reducing GBS-related infections, actually increased the incidence of ampicillin-resistant gram-negative neonatal sepsis with increasing mortality. Additionally, a positive vaginal test for GBS is not necessarily a reliable predictor of whether a newborn will develop a serious infection. On the other hand, another study found that GBS in term infants can also occur in women who were screened but tested negative for GBS.

Risks of GBS Screening

There are women who decline universal GBS testing, opting for the risk-based approach during labor. Universal prescribing of antibiotics for all GBS positive women, including those who are not considered high risk, exposes many mothers and babies to antibiotics. Concerns have been raised over the use of antibiotics and their potential contribution to antibiotic resistance in newborns, as well as allergic reactions (known anaphylaxis) in mothers. Common side effects of antibiotic use include yeast infections such as thrush in both mother and baby which can interfere with breastfeeding. The current medicine of choice is penicillin. In the past, other antibiotics such as amoxicillin were used; however, these are no longer used due to resistance. The prophylactic treatment has focused mainly on short-term effects regarding GBS, but researchers are now beginning to consider the long-term effects, although there is not yet any data on this.

Alternatives

Despite this information, there are women who decline the GBS testing or antibiotics altogether. Although there is not much research on alternatives to antibiotics, many midwives and alternative practitioners recommend the use of natural supplements that may help reduce the colonization of GBS in the vagina and boost the immune system. Be sure to discuss alternative treatments with your practitioner. Some women also choose to begin boosting the immune system prior to the GBS test which may help reduce or eliminate the colonization of GBS.

When a woman receives antibiotics for GBS, an IV will be placed, usually in the forearm. The infusion takes approximately 15 to 30 minutes. Since it is given every 4 hours, the IV itself is detachable, and can allow a laboring woman to move freely. Many home birth midwives offer IV antibiotics, thus GBS positive women can deliver at home, at a birth center, or in a hospital.

Although we may not know the long-term effects of antibiotics, we do know about the importance of the immune system—including the initial exposure to gut flora from mother to baby—so expectant mothers could consider preparing for the GBS testing ahead of time.

Prior to being tested for GBS, consider ways to help boost your immune system and avoid increased risks of GBS growth by avoiding unnecessary vaginal exams during late pregnancy as this exam can lead to early rupture of membranes. In general, eat well, get plenty of rest, participate in moderate exercise, and avoid overly stressful situations. Using alternative therapies to boost the immune system may help reduce or eliminate the vaginal colonization of GBS.

Although not backed up by scientific research, the following home remedies are used successfully by midwives. Consider taking one or more of the following immune boosters several weeks prior to GBS screening:

❀ Consider taking one or more of the following general immune strengtheners several weeks prior to GBS screening:

  ❀ Probiotics, orally and/or vaginally

  ❀ Immune supplements including echinacea, vitamin C, grapefruit seed extract, and colloidal silver

  ❀ Garlic is known for its antibacterial properties. Eat plenty of fresh garlic. In addition, insert a peeled and scored clove of garlic into the vagina for three nights prior to the test. Remove and discard it every morning. You will most likely taste the garlic in your mouth, not to worry!

  ❀ Insert plain, cultured yogurt vaginally twice per week

  ❀ Eat fermented foods including sauerkraut, yogurt, kefir, etc. (throughout pregnancy)

❀ For GBS-positive women in labor or those who are at higher risk for GBS infections, the Hibiclens (chlorhexidine) vaginal flush protocol is used by midwives for those who refuse antibiotic treatment. Hibiclens is an over-the-counter antiseptic and antimicrobial skin cleanser which has been shown to reduce GBS infection in newborns.

  ❀ Method: Prepare the 0.2% chlorhexidine solution by combining approximately 7cc (1½ teaspoons) Hibiclens (4% chlorhexidine solution) with 133 cc (½ cup plus 2 teaspoons) warm water. While reclining or sitting with hips elevated on several towels, slowly infuse the solution into the vagina under gentle pressure using a peri bottle. This can be done by the woman or any other person. Begin at onset of labor or rupture of membranes, repeating every 4 to 6 hours. Use the entire amount for each flush.

Gestational Diabetes (GD)

Testing for gestational diabetes (also known as gestational diabetes mellitus, GDM) is done routinely by most practitioners in pregnancy. Diabetes is a medical condition that occurs when the pancreas does not produce enough insulin (type 1 diabetes) or when the body is unable to use the insulin efficiently (type 2 diabetes). Following a meal, sugar and carbohydrates are converted into glucose in the blood. Insulin is a hormone which enables the body's cells to use the blood glucose as a source of energy for the body and the brain. During pregnancy, hormones secreted from the placenta minimize the effectiveness of mother's insulin in the body. As a result of this insulin resistance, the glucose is not properly utilized by the cells, leading to elevated blood sugar, called hyperglycemia. Gestational diabetes is found to occur in up to 7 percent of all pregnant women, usually in late pregnancy. Although gestational diabetes disappears after pregnancy, mothers are more at risk of diabetes type 2 (non–insulin dependent) in the future. It is also believed the extra amount of sugar can cause baby to become larger in utero, which can lead to potential complications at birth including difficult delivery, low blood sugar, breathing problems, and increase risk for obesity and type 2 diabetes in adulthood.

Glucose Challenge Test

It is not uncommon for the mother's blood sugar to increase after eating, or after the testing done by the healthcare provider, called the glucose challenge test. The glucose challenge test (GCT) is a routine screening test done for all women between the 24th and the 28th weeks of pregnancy. Although any woman can have gestational diabetes, risk factors include obesity, high blood pressure, family history of diabetes, exposure to pesticides, number of pregnancies (parity), and certain ethnic groups (Hispanic, African American, American Indian, or Asian).

The test is done in the morning after fasting from the night before. One hour after drinking a sugary solution called Glucola (50 gm glucose) your practitioner will take a blood sample to check blood sugar level (within a five-minute period). The results give an idea of how efficiently the body utilizes the sugar. At St. John Hospital and Medical Center, a study concluded that ingesting 28 jelly beans may serve as an alternative to Glucola (50 gm glucose). Many women do not tolerate the sweetness in the drink and this study found that the jelly beans were preferred by women compared to the 50 gm Glucola beverage.

For women who have an abnormal glucose challenge test (blood sugar value greater than 130 mg/dl to 140 mg/dl), there is the 3-hour glucose tolerance test (GTT) which is more definitive for diabetes. For the GTT, a fasting blood sugar is drawn before drinking a more concentrated Glucola drink (75 to 100 gm of glucose), and blood and urine are tested at intervals of 1 hour, 2 hours, and 3 hours. A reading of two abnormal values confirms gestational diabetes. Although not researched, some practitioners are known to use a more common sense approach by having the patient eat a meal for the test instead of the beverage.

Sample Diet for 1 Hour GTT:
 2 scrambled eggs (3 ounces)
 2 slices toast or English muffin
 2 pats butter or margarine
 8 ounces orange juice
 8 ounces whole milk
 1 cup coffee or tea (no sugar)

Considerations

Gestational diabetes is not diagnosed based on any complaints or symptoms, but rather on laboratory findings following the ingesting of a large amount of sugar. Because this test may offer information about the mother being more at risk of diabetes type 2 in the future, Dr. Michel Odent writes, "One might even claim that the only interest of glucose tolerance test in pregnancy is to identify a population at risk of developing a type 2 diabetes." Dr. Sarah Buckley believes that it would be normal for a mother's blood sugar to be higher in order to meet her growing baby's needs and functions. According to author Henci Goer, the original series of studies on the risks of high blood sugar and pregnancy were flawed. The research was originally conducted on a large group of pregnant women without any consideration of nutritional status or norms on blood glucose level in healthy well-nourished pregnant women. One of the concerns of diabetes and pregnancy is having a large baby (known as macrosomia). In the end, it was found that maternal weight was the most important predictor of having a big baby, not blood glucose. The link between GDM and bigger babies is clear; however, questions arise as to whether bigger babies are due in general to weight gain in pregnancy and/or obesity first, which then caused the GDM. A diagnosis of GDM increases the chance of being induced earlier than the baby is ready, because doctors become concerned about delivery of large babies.

Childbirth experts in the natural birth community consider gestational diabetes more as a finding of high blood sugar following the glucose tolerance test (GTT), rather than a disease because GDM resolves after the baby is born. According to Ina May Gaskin, the test is not reliable because 50 to 70 percent of women who are re-tested following an abnormal reading will have a different result than that from the first test, "The best evidence we have says there is no treatment for gestational diabetes, either with diet or with insulin that improves the outcomes for mothers or their babies. In short, the anxiety that is often produced by this test simply isn't worth the information gained from it."

With this information, it would clearly be ideal for an obese woman to lose weight before conceiving. Abnormal results of this test can be a cause of great anxiety, and in addition many women are not counseled properly and can be rushed into insulin therapy. According to Dr. Brewer, an obstetrician known for his pregnancy diet: "...thousands of pregnant women will be falsely diagnosed as diabetic and then be further mismanaged in terms of their nutritional needs."

In addition to diet, exercise has a beneficial effect on insulin sensitivity and improves the mother's blood sugar. In particular, research has shown that upper-arm exercise was significant and in some cases prevented the need for insulin. During my second pregnancy, my test showed that my blood sugars were border-line for gestational diabetes. My midwife had me fine-tune my diet and told me to begin upper-arm exercises...lots of them. It was during summer, so I spent more time in the swimming pool. The subsequent test came back normal. With all this contradictory information, not all practitioners perform routine testing for GDM except in cases of high risk. The best approach would be to focus on healthy lifestyle tips, which include proper nutrition, exercise, and rest—all of which are important for all pregnant women, no matter what their size (see Chapter 1 for additional lifestyle tips).

Rh Factor (RhoGAM)

Another routine blood test done in pregnancy is for the presence of Rh factor (Rhesus). Eighty-five percent of the population carries the red blood cell marker and is Rh-positive. If one does not have it, they are considered Rh-negative. The rationale for this screening test is that when a woman with Rh-negative blood is exposed to the Rh-positive blood of her baby, this could lead to complications. In general, the mother's blood does not mix with baby's blood. However, there are rare cases where this can happen, and it can lead to sensitization.

If a pregnant woman is Rh-negative and father is Rh-positive, the baby will most likely be Rh-positive. If both parents are Rh-negative, then the baby will be Rh-negative, and there is no concern for sensitization. When a mother with Rh-negative blood is exposed to baby's Rh factor, her blood can become sensitized and mount an attack against the baby's blood. This can lead to the breakdown of the baby's red blood cells, causing anemia, jaundice, or on rare occasions, a more severe case known as hemolytic disease in the newborn which could be fatal. Further blood tests, such as the Coombs tests (direct and indirect) are used to determine if a woman has become sensitized.

Risks for a mother becoming sensitized include blood transfusion, abortion, miscarriage, ectopic pregnancy, a traumatic accident to the belly, external version (for breech), episiotomy, and even after amniocentesis or CVS. This is rarely an issue in the first pregnancy as antibodies have not yet begun to develop, but is more important in subsequent pregnancies. Even routine cord clamping, a standard procedure in the medical model, can affect exposure. According to Dr. Sarah Buckley, immediately clamping the cord at the time of delivery traps the blood in the placenta (100 ml of blood) which is squeezed during third stage contractions (delivery of the placenta). At this point, the baby is already born; however the contractions can force baby's blood past the barrier and lead to mixing of the blood, known as fetal-maternal hemorrhage (FMH). FMH can lead to sensitization in the mother's blood, and can be reactivated in subsequent pregnancies if she is carrying an Rh-positive baby. Buckley writes about the emergence of FMH with the use of Pitocin induction (oxytocin) because the stronger uterine contractions can cause microfractures in the placental barrier, "The use of oxytocic drugs, either during labor or in third stage has been linked to an increased risk of FMH and blood group incompatibility problems." (See Chapter 3 for more information on cord clamping.)

Since the 1960s, pregnant women who are Rh-negative have been given an injection of Rh immunoglobulin (RhIg, also known as RhoGAM) that prevents mother's blood from forming antibodies in future pregnancies of women carrying Rh-positive babies. RhoGAM is routinely given to mothers at approximately 28 weeks of pregnancy. The shot lasts approximately 12 weeks, and is repeated within 72 hours of birth to mothers with Rh positive babies, in case there is any blood exposure.

Benefits of RhoGAM

If baby is Rh positive, RhoGAM can be given after baby's blood type is determined from a sample taken from the cord blood at the time of birth. RhoGAM is considered an effective shot and has reduced the number of complications and deaths from hemolytic disease. The shot is considered safe, according to the manufacturer.

Risks of RhoGAM

Use of RhoGAM is not completely without controversy. Questions arise regarding how much protection it provides, and for how long. RhoGAM is made from human blood plasma and there is the risk of infection. Although the risk is uncommon, it can occur as with any donor blood. Side effects to RhoGAM include local swelling inflammation at the site, skin rash, body aches, and on rare occasions, anaphylactic reaction such as hives. The standard RhoGAM preparation has contained the mercury compound, thimerosal. However, mercury-free RhoGAM is usually available, though it still contains preservatives. According to the manufacturer, "Animal studies have not been conducted. Available evidence suggests that Rho (D) immune globulin administration during pregnancy does not harm the fetus or affect future pregnancies." According to birth experts who advocate a gentle, undisturbed and natural birth process with minimal intervention and time allowance for the placenta to separate, there is usually no mixing of blood between mother and baby. This means an Rh-negative mother would not become sensitized. Traumatic and difficult births increase the likelihood for sensitization. However, practitioners have no precise way to know.

Considerations

In weighing the risks and benefits of receiving RhoGAM, some women have elected to not have the 28th week shot routinely, and instead choose the mercury-free RhoGAM shot within 72 hours of giving birth if baby is Rh-positive, or if there is a high risk event during pregnancy. According to midwife Ina May Gaskin,

"The problem with routine prescription of prenatal RhoGAM is that many babies who are Rh-negative like their mothers will be exposed to the drug, and there has been no systematic study of the long-term effects of this product in babies."

Vaccinations during Pregnancy

Vaccinations such as Tdap (Tetanus, Diphtheria, and Pertussis) and the flu shot are recommended during pregnancy. The Tdap is recommended because it offers protection for the newborn against pertussis (whooping cough). Whooping cough occurs in both children and adults, but is considered a more serious infection in infants. The vaccination is given to pregnant women (and their family members, including visiting grandparents) because it can be passed from adults to children. The flu shot (from the inactivated virus, not the live virus nose spray type) is recommended during the flu season, from October to March.

Having these vaccines during pregnancy is considered safe by such organizations as the Centers for Disease Control. However, according to Barbara Loe Fisher of the National Vaccine Information Center, "Drug companies did not test the safety and effectiveness of giving influenza or Tdap vaccine to pregnant women before the vaccines were licensed in the United States and there is almost no data on inflammatory or other biological responses to these vaccines that could affect pregnancy and birth outcomes." In the federal Vaccine Injury Compensation Program (VICP), the most compensated claim from complications (including death) is from vaccines containing pertussis, and the flu shot is the second most common claim. This is a difficult choice for many women because of the pressure from many healthcare practitioners, and Barbara Loe Fisher urges parents to request that the doctor show them the information about the vaccines, including the science behind them. From there, you can make an informed choice.

The Wonderment of Childbirth: Natural Birth and the Medical Approach

The Normal Birth Process

During my first pregnancy, like most women, I anticipated childbirth with excitement, apprehension, and fear. I wondered what it would feel like, and questioned whether I could handle the pain. I would remind myself that birth is not an illness or a disease, and rarely is it an emergency. Birth is a perfectly natural experience. In fact, most births, if allowed to progress free from intervention, are absolutely normal. I thought of our maternal heritage, generation upon generation of expectant mothers, just like me. Realizing that every human being is born from a mother, my confidence began to grow. So many women experience childbirth, and so can I. In fact, women are exquisitely designed for pregnancy, and our bodies know how to birth!

In order for humans to walk upright with two limbs (bipedalism) the pelvis is narrower compared to other mammals. Yet the pelvis is also the passageway during birth, and must be able to accommodate the baby—head, shoulders, and all. Doctors are taught that human birth is more difficult compared to other mammals, due to the large brain size of the baby and the narrow pelvis of the mother. However, homo sapiens have adapted to allow for normal birth; otherwise the species would not have survived. For delivery, several mechanisms occur which allow for flexibility from both mother and baby. Before birth, the hormone *relaxin* softens the pelvic ligaments, allowing the mother's pelvis to widen—even 4 mm can make a big difference! With changes in blood flow and nutrients to the baby, a pregnant mother's body can also adapt to the size of the fetus. The baby's head is comprised of skull bone plates which move and slide over each other, allowing the baby to descend through the pelvis. This is accomplished through a mastery of twists and rotations during delivery. It helps that human infants are also born smaller than other mammalian newborns; they are also more immature and helpless.

For natural birth pioneer Dr. Michel Odent, the normal birth process is about "not thinking too much." In fact, the primary obstacle that human beings must overcome is not the fact that the homo sapiens' pelvis is small or the baby's head too large, but the hindrance of the intellectual brain (neocortex) in the mother (and in her support team). Birth is a primal experience; it demands a woman's intuition and instinct. It is not meant to be a logical or rational event. Yet, we live in a culture that is intellectually predominant. Yes, we can engage our intellect in preparation, for example through reading, discussions, and birth classes. But on the *birth day*, the requisite for a normal birth to proceed is when the laboring woman is given the permission to be herself, undisturbed. Her thinking, worrying brain—the neocortex—is at rest, allowing the birthing hormones to be released uninhibited. She is able to behave and move instinctively without reserve. The decreased activity of the brain also allows her to more easily work through the contractions, enabling her to tolerate and surrender to the pain and discomfort. A woman who feels comfortable in her birthing space feels free to grunt, yell, scream, and move freely from all-fours to circular rocking motions—all of which she would not do in her civilized life. When asked for advice in helping give birth, midwife Ina May Gaskin says, "Let your monkey do it!" This means letting the animal primate within each of us do the work of labor because monkeys are not self-conscious; they are not concerned with what they look like, how they act, or how they move. They embrace the ancient wisdom of a woman's body, an essential part of childbirth, while avoiding neocortex activity which halts and inhibits labor. In other words, do not do anything during labor that stimulates the brain; for example, avoid bright lights, noise, everyday conversation, and frequent interruptions. Also, turn off cell phone ringers and remove all clocks and watches.

When our ancestors lived in villages, many women would have been at births, or at least have been familiar with the process. As the birth world became more medicalized and less familial (and less *familiar*), for many women the only exposure to childbirth are those portrayed by the media which consists of a caricature of a laboring woman out of control, tethered to the bed in stirrups, screaming in agony. However, for many natural birth experts, an undisturbed birth is viewed as an ecstatic experience, where pleasure and pain are but two sides of the same coin. There are various adjectives to describe childbirth, but the word *ecstatic* is a far cry from the television version. We have been brainwashed into believing that birth is a horribly painful experience which needs to be treated as a medical emergency waiting to happen rather than as a normal process. According to many natural birth experts, birth can be a pleasurable experience. When a woman is allowed the opportunity to birth in a secure and uninterrupted place, the possibility for transforming a painful experience into a euphoric one can unfold. According to Dr. Sarah Buckley, "Giving birth in ecstasy: this is our birthright and our body's intent. Mother Nature, in her wisdom, prescribes birthing hormones that take us outside our usual state so that we can be transformed on every level as we enter motherhood. This exquisite hormonal orchestration unfolds optimally when birth is undisturbed, enhancing safety for both mother and baby." For many people, ecstasy conjures up references to sexuality or a higher state from drugs or the spiritual realm—an *out of this world* feeling. These comments are not unusual following an undisturbed labor as many women report a feeling that is indescribable.

Known to be one of the best kept secrets about birth, up to 21 percent of women surveyed had experienced an orgasm during childbirth. It is not uncommon to witness caresses, kisses, and deep affection between partners during labor. According to Dr. Christiane Northrup, birth is a sensual experience and the same organs and intricate hormonal system responsible for delivery of the baby were the ones present at conception nine months earlier. Because of the parallels, when possible, the birthing space should be similar to the lovemaking one: intimate, private, sacred, and serene.

Birth Hormones: The Agony and Ecstasy

The limbic system is part of the mammalian brain which controls behaviors related to emotions, survival, and sexual behavior. According to Dr. Michel Odent, hormones are secreted from this evolutionary primitive brain structure known as the *love cocktail*: oxytocin, beta endorphins, adrenaline, and prolactin. These hormones affect the body as well as behavior, and play a large role in humankind.

Oxytocin: The Cuddle Hormone

Oxytocin, known as the cuddle hormone, is responsible for romantic feelings, love, trust, and monogamy, as well as the mother-child bond. Released from the pituitary gland in the brain, it plays an important role in orgasm for both sexes; and birth it helps with dilation of the cervix, aids in labor and delivery of baby and placenta, and controls bleeding in the postpartum period. During breastfeeding it also plays a role in the "let down" of milk. Oxytocin is one of the hormones responsible for the elation mother can experience following birth as she touches and sees her baby for the first time. Research has shown that children who are autistic have lower levels of oxytocin. (See "Inducing Labor" on page 89 for a discussion on pitocin.)

Endorphins: The Hormonal Pain Killer

Endorphins, also produced by the pituitary gland, resemble opiates and work as a natural analgesic. Endorphins provide us with a feeling of well-being and pleasure that is released during such experiences as strenuous exercise, pain, and orgasm. The release of this natural morphine-like hormone helps to ease a mother's pain threshold while giving birth. In effect, the release of beta endorphins during childbirth is nature's pain medication, and one that does not deleteriously affect mother or baby. During childbirth the beta endorphins allow the mother to be transformed, altering her state of consciousness and allowing her to transcend the pain and discomfort. It is not uncommon for women to say afterward that they felt as if they were *on another planet*, comments similar to being on opiates.

Adrenaline (Epinephrine): The Fight or Flight Response

Adrenaline and noradrenaline (epinephrine and norepinephrine), known as the catecholamines (CA), are secreted by the adrenal gland above the kidneys. They regulate heart rate, blood flow, and respiration. This hormone is secreted in situations that require a *fight* or *flight* response. From drinking coffee to thrill-seeking activities, there are people known as "adrenaline junkies" who savor the *rush*. Adrenaline is also released in stressful situations, such as during road rage in a traffic jam. In nature, when a laboring animal in the wild senses danger, adrenaline is secreted, and it stops her contractions allowing her to flee to a safe place. In delivery, there is a normal CA surge released at the end of labor, called the fetal ejection reflex. It is also secreted by the infant in preparing the lungs for breathing and increasing blood flow, all of which support survival. The CA surge also accounts for the initial alert time that occurs at birth, allowing for bonding between mother and baby. On the other hand, when a woman does not feel protected or safe, too much is secreted. When this occurs, high CA levels inhibit oxytocin which can lead to prolonged labor or can shut down labor altogether.

Prolactin: The Mothering Hormone

Prolactin, the breastfeeding hormone, begins its production during pregnancy. Also known as the mothering hormone, prolactin also aids with nesting, which prepares for the bonding between mother and baby. Especially in the first few months of life, it helps mother with relaxation, sleep, and patience.

From a chicken laying an egg to a horse birthing its foal, we can learn from other species. A birthing animal needs a quiet secluded space. She must be free of unnecessary interruptions and able to move in various positions, as she feels. So it is with humans. A woman in labor is literally opening herself to new life. She is vulnerable and needs to feel safe, with privacy, to labor. When relaxed, her cervix opens. Activities such as the drive to the hospital, the admission process, and visits from nurses and doctor can trigger the release of adrenaline and close the cervix, thus impeding the birth process. When possible, it is best for the mother to be proactive and address any concerns ahead of time, which may help diminish her anticipation. For some women, taking the hospital tour and doing admission paperwork beforehand may help minimize undue stress during labor.

The medical model of care can interfere with the normal flow of birth hormones. For this reason, the use of standard medications during labor and delivery are meant to be reserved for extreme conditions and medical emergencies. When used for emergencies, many lives have been saved. However, success has also led to excessive use of interventions such as medications. The medical model uses interventions for most women, most of whom are not considered high risk. Thus, it creates a situation of a viscous cycle in which the interventions necessitate the need for more interventions. Ultimately it becomes a slippery slope, drastically changing a woman's birth plan for a natural and unmedicated birth.

The Stages of Childbirth: Birth Cues and Clues

Childbirth is a different experience for each woman, as well as for each delivery. Labor and delivery is a holistic experience in that it will challenge you—physically, mentally, and emotionally. Physically, labor is a series of muscle contractions that dilate the cervix allowing baby to be pushed out of the womb into the birth canal. Contractions can be felt in the belly, pelvis, hips, and lower back. The frequency, power, and length of contractions also vary. Labor for first-time mothers typically lasts approximately 12 to 18 hours, although some labors seem to be ongoing for days. If this is not your first baby you can expect labor to be quicker, although that is not always the case.

Sometimes labor is drawn-out, slows down, or stops altogether. If this occurs after18 to 24 hours, it is known as "prolonged labor" or "failure to progress." This could be due to the position of the baby, weak contractions, improper position of the mother, or stressful circumstances causing a woman to "close up" (see "Birth Hormones" on page 64). The stages of childbirth are unique to each woman, yet also present characteristic signposts. Each stage of birth includes physical qualities as well as emotional signposts, the latter come from the Bradley Method. I enjoyed my birth class and encourage couples to attend a comprehensive course that reviews these stages of childbirth and a lot more. With the right teacher, the information and experience can be as helpful for your partner as it is for you.

Resting in Between Contractions

During labor there is much focus on the contractions. As the stages of labor progress, so do the contractions. However, in between contractions are the rest times. These quiet times allow you to regroup, recharge, and relax. Dozing off between contractions is not uncommon, as it gathers strength for the next contraction. For this reason, it is important for you to have a birth space to labor undisturbed, without questions and conversation so you can rest during contractions.

First Stage of Labor: Labor

The first stage of childbirth is the *labor* itself, when your cervix ultimately becomes fully dilated, which will then lead you to the 2nd stage of labor, known as delivery or the pushing stage. The first stage is divided into three parts: early labor, active labor, and transition.

Early Labor: "The excitement of it all…"

Following what may be days or weeks of occasional pre-labor contractions, early labor is marked by contractions that become more regular, occurring every 5 to 20 minutes and lasting 30–45 seconds. In this stage the cervix opens from 0 to 3 cm. Early labor typically lasts up to 8–12 hours duration for a first time mother. This is the longer stage of labor, and the easiest. You may need to stop and breathe through a contraction, which may feel like pressure or cramping. The contractions at this stage are from mild to moderate intensity. You may have diarrhea, or notice a blood-tinged vaginal discharge, which is probably your mucus plug that has been released from the cervical opening.

Emotional Cues: Emotionally, you may feel excited, happy, and even a little nervous in anticipation that this is "the day." During early labor (up to 3–4 cm), you are usually able to talk during a contraction. You can appear excited, happy, and all smiles, between contractions as you anticipate birth. Unless medically contraindicated, a warm bath or shower can be relaxing. If you are giving birth at a hospital or birth center, it is best to avoid the urge to go to the hospital too early (unless directed to). Stay at home, as it is early in the game.

What to Do (for Coaches): Distract her with other things besides labor and avoid being focused on the clock. Keep it simple: finish up last minute tasks, take a walk, go to a restaurant, and even visit with friends. Enjoy yourselves, watch a silly movie. Eating and drinking are important at this stage. Intuitively, she may have certain cravings, but it is best to keep the food simple, with small portions. Eat when hungry. Naps are good and if it is bedtime, try to sleep.

Active Labor: "This is serious stuff..."

As you move to the next phase, known as active labor, your contractions become longer and stronger, coming every 3 to 4 minutes and lasting 40 to 60 seconds (or longer). The cervix opens now from 3 to 7 cm, and active labor typically lasts 3 to 5 hours.

Emotional Cues: Your mood is now more serious and focused as contractions require more concentration. Vocalizing through the contractions may begin during the active phase as a way to stay relaxed and open. You are less chatty and less modest. You probably do not want to be disturbed, but may appreciate comfort measures from a back rub to pressure points.

What to Do (for Coaches): As she nears 6 cm dilated, she will no longer be hungry, but it is important for her to stay hydrated. Offer a few sips of a healthy drink in between contractions Movement and changing position are important to help baby navigate its way through the birth canal. Some healthcare providers use the 4-1-1 rule as a guideline of when to leave for the birthplace: when contractions are 4 minutes apart, lasting one minute in length, and continuing for over one hour.

Transition: "I give up; I doubt I can do this..."

How wonderful! You are almost there. But, it is tough. This is the most difficult part, but also the shortest. Transition lasts 30 minutes to 2 hours. In this stage, the contractions come every 2 to 3 minutes and last 60 to 90 seconds. Contractions are strong and may have double peaks. Here the cervix opens to 7 to 10 cm which means by the end of transition, you are fully dilated and ready to push. Physically, you may become shaky, nauseated, and chilled. At this stage vomiting, burping, hiccupping, and having hot and cold flashes are not uncommon.

Emotional Cues: This is a common time for you to feel defeated, that you cannot go on anymore. Self-doubt sets in. You are ready to give up the desire you had for a natural birth and may want to take the drugs. As labor progresses it becomes more difficult to speak. By 5 to 7 cm, the sounds go from open vowels or a hum to becoming louder, repetitive, and staccato. At this stage it is impossible to talk through a contraction. Your mood shifts as you enter the realm of the "birth space." You can become easily irritated by trivial interruptions and conversation.

What to Do (for Coaches): As part of the support team, this is precisely the time when she needs to be reassured to keep going just like a marathon runner who is at the final 3 miles. If it is appropriate, you can remind her, "You are almost there. You are doing an awesome job." This is the stage that is most mishandled in the hospital. It is very important now to have a good birth team doula or a midwife who will praise her because they know she is almost finished. In addition to positive reinforcement, she also needs to be able to feel free to moan, groan, and move about. Do not bother her with questions. Yet, she may ask for touch and pressure. By this stage, the midwife has arrived for a home birth or mother has already arrived at her birthplace, such as the hospital or birth center.

It is important to remember that stages of labor drift and overlap, one into another. During my labors, I was less concerned about the numerical details of my contractions and more focused on surrendering to them, one at a time. I couldn't wait for labor to be finished, and to meet my baby!

Second Stage of Labor: Pushing

Once fully dilated, transition has passed and contractions ease up a little bit. Now marks the beginning of delivery, known as the pushing stage. During this stage, contractions last 60 seconds but with a break of 3 to 5 minutes in between. Pushing can be for 30 minutes to 2 hours. At this time, you may feel more rejuvenated and able to speak. The pushing stage for my first baby was three hours long. For my second child, it was a few minutes of pushing, with ease. For some women the urge to push is involuntary, while for others requires encouragement and guidance from the practitioner. As with having a bowel movement, most women will hold their breath while pushing. After I had pushed for several hours, I will never forget when my midwife told me, "You can lift your baby out now!"

Note: It is not uncommon to hear that a woman is ready to push but, because the doctor has not arrived at the hospital, she is told by the nurses to cross her legs and "Stop, don't push!" Being told to stop a natural urge can be stressful for both mother and baby. According to birth instructor Kathy Killebrew, "When this force within is powerful, it needs to be worked *with*, not against, nor ignored. It is cruel to ask a woman to go against everything her body wants to do. Perhaps for some it is possible to hold back before the urge is irresistibly strong, but for those who want to push, it's painful to hold back! I have encouraged expectant parents in my class to ask for the on-call doctor rather than holding their babies in."

Third Stage of Labor: Delivery of the Placenta

Amazing—baby is born! Intense contractions cease, for the most part. Still there are smaller contractions that help detach your placenta from the uterine wall allowing it to ultimately be expelled from the birth canal; this is known as the third stage.

If everything has gone smoothly, your baby is on your chest where everyone can rejoice and baby can begin breastfeeding. As new parents, you are now faced with joys, challenges, and more decisions to make. Mother and baby should stay together, unless absolutely medically needed. A new chapter begins. (See my book *Natural Baby and Childcare* for advice on the next 20 years.)

More on Birth...

No matter where you choose to birth, it is important that you find your comfort zone. The ideal space should feel safe and private; somewhere you can feel comfortable surrendering through a contraction. With low-pitched groans, grunts and moans, sounding allows your body to release and give in to the contractions. High-pitched sounds are more tensing to the body. As you move to transition and full dilation, it is not uncommon for you to feel as if you cannot continue. You may even exclaim, "I can't do this anymore!" In an optimal birth setting, your support team should be familiar with these birth markers and know to look for these signs, as they offer information about where you are in your birth progress.

The Bradley Method offers guidance on the emotional signposts to look for as women move through the different stages of labor. The beginning of labor is marked with excitement. As contractions become more active (and more serious), so does your mood. Ultimately there comes a point where self-doubt creeps in, and you feel you need pain medications, even though your birth plan says otherwise.

These signposts are not meant to offer guidelines that are "hard and fast," rules, but which are rather individual and unique to each woman and each labor. Moving through stages can be encouraging because it lets you know that changes are in progress. When a woman desires to spend as much time as possible laboring at home, these signposts can offers signals that can mean stay at home now, or it is time to go to the birthplace.

Vocalization and the Sphincter Law

A very helpful exercise I learned from my birth instructor that I was able to apply during my first labor was vocalizing my way through each contraction. With a low-toned hum, moan, or groan, my throat opened, relaxing my neck, chest, and pelvis. In doing so, I felt as if I were riding with the wave, as opposed to being crushed by a tsunami.

My instructor taught us comfort techniques to avoid tensing the body, which only hinders labor. Vocalization is an unstructured breathing technique that, by allowing the breath to flow, provides for oxygenation to mother and baby, promotes relaxation, and distracts mother by encouraging her to focus on breath. With vocalization, not all sounds are created equal—especially in labor. A high-pitched scream or squeal is not only deafening but constricts the throat and the lower body. On the other hand, a low-pitched sound calms the body, allowing the cervix to relax and open. As contractions increase, so may the volume of the sound. At births, I have found this technique useful when a mother is struggling with contractions. Birth coaches can gently make the sound as a reminder to mother, and she will often imitate. In addition, noises such as chants, mantras, or grunts like those of a weight lifter can also be used. As my instructor reminded us, "Open throat, open cervix."

The cervix is the neck of the womb. As part of the lower end of the uterus, the cervix connects the uterus to the vagina, or birth canal. It is an opening which permits passage of menstrual blood or sperm, as well as a baby. During labor the cervix dilates large enough to accommodate the baby. Famed midwife Ina May Gaskin coined the term, *sphincter law*, as the cervix acts in a similar fashion to sphincters in the body, such as the urethra and anus. The latter are comprised of ring like muscles or fibers which maintain a constriction at an opening or orifice, but are also capable of relaxing as needed for normal bodily functions such as urinating and defecating. According to Gaskin, sphincters are "shy," they contract and dilate optimally in seclusion and privacy. So it is with babies. The cervix is like a sphincter in that its ability to open and close is not done at will, and does not respond well under pressure. During labor, the cervix opens, allowing passage of the baby into the birth canal. However, if a woman is interrupted, causing her to feel inhibited, guarded, or self-conscious, a surge of adrenaline is released which reverses its motion, closing the cervix (see "Birth Hormones" on page 64).

In many ways, the opening of the birth canal mirrors the state of the woman, an example of the mind-body connection. From an early age, we are taught social norms and customs around sphincter control for common everyday bodily functions. In other words, most people are more comfortable urinating, defecating, and passing gas in private. And so it is with childbirth. According to Gaskin, the inhibition factor in birth is one of the important reasons why, in traditional cultures, women delivered the babies. Tying this idea in with techniques such as vocalization, "The state of relaxation of the mouth and jaw is directly correlated to the ability of the cervix, vagina, and anus to open to full capacity." The ease of opening of the birth canal which is not under our control is facilitated by the voluntary opening and relaxing of the throat with breath, laughter, and voice following the adage, "as above, so below."

FROM THE DOCTOR'S DESK

Suzanne invited a dozen friends to come and witness her third home birth. Her labor would progress and then stall, in a stop-and-start fashion. The midwife sensed that having too many people in the room was causing a "hiccup" in her progress, and asked everyone to leave other than dad. She delivered shortly thereafter.

Perineal Massage

For the weeks prior to my birth I soaked in a basin of raspberry leaf tea, and did perineal massage. I attribute all of these measures as being helpful in avoiding not only an episiotomy but also any tears with my deliveries of my boys who were 8½ lbs (3.86 kg). My birth classes were helpful, but it was never the same as the birth itself. Each birth was different too. Through patience, and the olive oil from our kitchen, our baby's head crowned and ultimately delivered—without a stitch.

The research on perineal massage is mixed and contradictory. One study showed that perineal massage during pushing did not have any effect on an intact perineum. However, perineal massage conducted before birth has some benefit in reducing damage to the perineum, especially in women 30 years and older. Intuitively, I felt in accordance with William and Martha Sears, authors of the *Birth Book*, who wrote, "The better you prepare your perineal tissues for the stretching of birth, the less they will tear, and the better they will heal." I also learned from my midwives and birth teacher that by massaging the perineum in the weeks leading up to birth, women become more familiar with sensations in the perineum. As a result, one can relax more into the familiar stinging and burning sensation (known as the "ring of fire") during crowning.

Perineal massage is done by your partner or yourself. Sit comfortably (in bed, in a chair, or on a toilet) with legs apart propped up in a semi-squat position. With clean hands, lubricate using a natural oil (such as almond oil, olive oil, or water-soluble lubricating jelly) and gently insert thumbs approximately 1 to 1 ½ inches inside the vagina. Press downwards toward the rectum on the perineum with a "U" shaped motion in the lower part of the vagina. Gently stretch, hold, and massage the tissue for at least 5 minutes at least every other day. Initially you will experience a burning sensation which will decrease with subsequent sessions. Begin after week 36. Discuss with your practitioner before beginning.

Ring of Fire

Similar to many others, as a first-time mother, my pushing (the second stage) with my first child was much longer than my second birth. The first birth was 3 hours, compared to what seemed like only three pushes for the second birth. Their personalities are as different as their births.

During the second stage of labor, mother works to push out the baby. When the baby's head crowns, it stretches the perineum and opens the vagina. It is common to feel a burning and stinging sensation, this is known as the "ring of fire." At this moment, the midwife or obstetrician will help guide mother: sometimes encouraging her to push, and other times to refrain from pushing. In our home birth, our midwife soaked small towels in the hot water my husband had ready for her, and gently placed the warm compresses to help soften the tissue of the perineum during delivery. In addition to the warmth, she used olive oil for massage and lubrication.

Discuss perineal massage with your healthcare provider. Consider performing it daily, beginning in the last month of pregnancy (week 36 and onward). This can be done by yourself or with your partner.

Comfort Measures during Labor: Nonmedical Relief

Empower Births is an acronym that I learned in my birth class, and which is meant to be used by both birth coach and the laboring woman. Originated from the Perinatal Education Associates (Birthsource.com), the significance behind each word can be applied individually to each woman. Make it your own.

E—Encouragement: A woman needs encouragement, praise, and reassurance. Avoid negative comments. Emotions can influence labor either way.

M—Massage: Light touch, stroking and counter pressure, and acupressure points (see below) can greatly aid a woman in labor. On the other hand, sometimes she does not want to be touched at all. Some women like pressure on the back. Try rolling a beverage can or the pressure points for the Double Hip Squeeze (with mother leaning forward, place hands on fleshy part of her buttocks, and press in toward the center). Follow her cues.

P—Position: Change position during labor every 30 to 45 minutes. Baby's descent and position is facilitated by movement including squatting, walking, lunges, slow dancing, swaying, using a birth ball, pelvic rocking, and more. Get creative. Try leaning over the birth ball and swaying. Rotating positions helps turn baby into an optimal position.

O—Open Mind: Flexibility in both mind and body are important. Sometimes our labors progress differently than we anticipated. Be open minded to options and choices.

W—Walking (and Movement): Walking during pregnancy and labor are important for optimizing baby's position in the birth canal, but can also help relieve discomfort. If possible, some women also appreciate a gentle walk outdoors during labor. Use a birth ball during pregnancy, labor, and beyond.

E—Empty Bladder and the Potty: A full bladder can get in the way. Try to urinate every hour. If mom is not able to urinate for more than a couple of hours, she may need straight catheterization. Many women appreciate sitting on the toilet as one of the good labor positions with the following benefits: upright position (uses gravity), encourages urination, facilitates bearing down, and relaxes perineum. Sitting on the toilet can also help her to position herself bent forward or arched backward. Keep pillows nearby, and try placing the feet on stools to open the pelvis and simulate squatting. Being on a toilet also encourages an atmosphere of privacy.

R—Refreshments: Childbirth requires stamina and energy. In early labor, light food that can be easily digested is crucial. Fluids are important throughout labor. Take 3 sips in between contractions especially during active labor, transition, and pushing. Water, coconut water, and natural sports drinks (such as Recharge®) with honey sticks are popular.

B—Breathing: Breathing is important as it brings oxygen to mother and baby. With pain and discomfort, the body wants to tense and stop breathing. For this reason, it is important to release the jaw and the face, and surrender with the breath. There are numerous childbirth education organizations that teach breathing techniques that many mothers have found helpful.

I—Imagery: It is said that birth is a mental experience. Mental imagery gives the woman's mind something to do. Some women respond well to images of being in a peaceful place, usually outside in nature. Others appreciate images of the cervix opening and melting around baby's head. Or try reciting nursery rhymes or bible verses. There is no single correct way to engage the mind.

R—Relaxation: When a woman can let go and relax, her labor progresses more smoothly and she experiences less pain. As labor progresses, vocalizing with deep moans and groans allows the body to surrender to the contractions. Even the goal of pain medicine is to help her relax.

T—Trust: A woman's body is designed to give birth, naturally. When a woman is provided with the right environment which includes the ability to move about freely, and is encouraged to trust in her body's internal wisdom, most women will be able to give birth without interventions and medication.

H—Honor the Process: Giving birth to new life is a process to be respected and honored.

S—Surroundings: A woman should feel as comfortable as possible during labor, and the ambiance is important. Animals typically go to a dark quiet place to birth, and so should we. Private, peaceful surroundings are important. Consider altering the lighting, sounds, and smells in the room. Dim lights are usually preferable to bright lights. Candles are not allowed in the hospital but some women appreciate a string of lights placed in the room. Be sure to keep the clock covered during labor.

. . .

Heat: Warm baths and showers can be soothing and relaxing. Some women appreciate a hot water bottle or heated rice sock on the groin or back. Fill a cotton sock (not synthetic) with dry rice (1½–2 lbs). Tie the open end of the sock. Heat in a microwave oven for 2–3 minutes. Place the sock on the back, side, or anywhere she wants. This will stay warm for 30 minutes. Bring the sock to the hospital, as it can be heated in a microwave.

Warm Water—Bathing and Birthing: The idea of soaking in a warm tub during labor or during birth is appealing to many women. While sitting in a warm tub, the body is more buoyant which allows for easier movement and changes in position. Not to mention that the water is soothing and relaxing and offers comfort, which optimizes her birth hormones of endorphins (natural pain relievers) and lessens the stress hormones. Warm water also allows the perineum to become more elastic, which may decrease tears. Water immersion can lessen the discomfort and allow for more efficient contractions, as well as lowering mother's blood pressure if due to anticipation. Also because being in a tub is an enclosed space, it gives mother more of a feeling of privacy. It becomes easier for her to lose her inhibitions and surrender to the labor experience. According to Dr. Michel Odent, director of the first underwater birthing facility in the West (France), being in the tub during labor accelerated the first stage of dilation while reducing the pain.

Water birth originally emerged from the midwifery model of birth and is now finding popularity in some hospitals and obstetrical medical settings. Based on the idea that the baby has lived in an amniotic fluid sac, being born into a similar environment can be a more gentle, less stressful transition at birth. Babies do not take their first breath until they come up for air. They stay oxygenated underwater through the umbilical cord. Tubs can be easily rented for labor use. Although most women are told to avoid water immersion if their water has broken, it is permitted once active labor has begun.

Cold: Some women may feel warm during labor and will instead appreciate cold applications. Rolling a soda can on the back can be soothing and cool. Make sure to keep some in your birth kit. Some women like an ice pack on the back. During my second labor I relied on a cold washcloth which I rubbed on my face and belly during each contraction—it was my greatest comfort!

Aromatherapy: A study which examined the use of ten essential oils (in a carrier oil) administered either on the skin or via inhalation, found that chamomile and clary sage especially were effective in alleviating labor pain. This suggests that aromatherapy can be effective in reducing maternal anxiety, fear and/or pain during labor. Aromatherapy can also be placed in a spray bottle or in a bowl.

Labor Companions, People and Visitors: The presence of doula is known to reduce the need and use of pain medication. Although having our male partners by our side is desirable, it does not seem to have the same medicinal effect as having an experienced woman (see "The Role of the Father" in Chapter 4). If anyone in the room is interfering with mother, they should be gently asked to leave. Beforehand, let others know that because this is a new experience, you do not know how you will respond and they should not be offended if you need your space. Note: You have the right to ask for a different nurse as well.

Delayed Cord Clamping

In the womb, the baby is sustained by nourishment and oxygen she receives from the umbilical cord which is connected to mother's placenta. The average length of the cord is 50 to 60 cm (20–23 in). At the time of birth, the blood continues to flow from the placenta to baby, until it is clamped or stops flowing on its own. The clamp is placed with a plastic clip close to the umbilical stump, and the remainder is cut (this is not painful). Ultimately the stump gives way to the belly button! At my first birth, we gave the honor of cutting my son's cord to my friend Sherilyn, who was pregnant at the time.

In the birth world, the optimal timing for clamping the cord has become a topic of debate. In the medical model, most practitioners were trained for "early clamping," as defined as clamping the umbilical cord usually less than a minute after birth. There is a commonly held belief in the obstetrical world that there is little or no benefit in delaying cord clamping and that waiting may lead to complications. Obstetrician Dr. Nicholas Fogelson from the USC School of Medicine states, "We are the only species that clamps the cord. In the past, baby was born and put on the breast. Doctors clamp the cord probably because it is convenient, and most do it routinely without thinking about it." Doctors are taught that delayed cord clamping, also known as placental transfusion, gives the baby too much blood. Although doctors in past centuries such as Erasmus Darwin (1731–1802), grandfather of Charles Darwin who knew about the importance of cord blood, wrote, "Another thing very injurious to the child is the tying and cutting of the navel string too soon—which should always be left till the child has not only repeatedly breathed but till all pulsations in the cord cease. As otherwise, the child is much weaker than it ought to be, a portion of the blood being left in the placenta which ought to have been in the child."

Allowing the cord to cease pulsating on its own only takes about 3 minutes, sometimes longer. Yet, studies have shown that the extra blood volume which comes from delaying until the flow from placenta to baby has ceased, is beneficial for the infant, particularly in infants who do not have access to good nutrition or are prone to severe anemia. Doctors are also taught that delayed clamping causes an increased risk of jaundice and harmful levels of increased blood volume in the baby. The connection between delayed cord clamping and increased jaundice in newborns is not substantiated by research. Bilirubin levels, which lead to jaundice, have been shown to not be altered by the timing of cord clamping. Premature clamping of the cord traps the blood in the placenta, and can lead to sensitizing mother's blood if she is Rh negative (see "Rh Factor" in Chapter 2). The increased blood volume means that more oxygen reaches the cells. In addition, although obstetricians believe there is an increased risk of mother bleeding after birth if the cord clamping is delayed, researchers found no evidence to support this. The medical profession is beginning to listen to the studies which show many health advantages in waiting. According to ACOG, reviews have suggested the importance of delaying cord clamping in premature infants because of the associated benefits of increased blood volume, less need for transfusion, and less incidence of intracranial hemorrhage. For term infants it is recognized that the benefits of waiting to clamp lowers frequency of anemia.

Benefits of Delayed Cord Clamping

Allowing the cord to stop pulsating and empty on its own provides up to 40 percent more blood volume (100 cc) for the baby. This substantially increases the newborn's blood volume and is optimal for the health of the baby's transition to life by increasing her hemoglobin and iron stores. Studies have shown that delaying cord clamping by 2 minutes increased a child's iron reserve by 27 to 47 mg, equivalent to 1 to 2 months worth of iron requirements and this increase is a factor in preventing iron deficiency in the first 6 months of life.

All in all, studies show that early clamping, which is widely used by obstetricians, is not justifiable. It seems sensible to delay cord clamping rather than intervene against the inherent wisdom of the human body. According to the World Health Organization, the flow of blood is likely self-regulated by the infant and there is evidence that the newborn is able to adjust to the increase in blood volume and viscosity. It is important to discuss this issue with your healthcare provider ahead of time.

Cord Blood Banking

Expectant couples are also faced with the decision of whether to store their baby's cord blood. Umbilical cord blood is rich in stem cells that may be used in the treatment of diseases later on including blood disorders, cancer, genetic diseases, and more. Banking the cord blood does not always mean it could be used in cases of the treatment of disease. It is an expensive venture, and it is not clear how long the blood can be successfully stored. Chances are remote that your child will use it, and for many practitioners the benefits do not outweigh the costs. Many medical organizations are not convinced of the benefits of storing cord blood. Cord blood collection requires collecting as much cord blood as is available, which requires early clamping of the cord. As described above, clamping of the cord too early deprives the newborn this extra blood, which is optimal for baby's hemoglobin and her health. In Dr. Sarah Buckley's book, *Gentle Birth, Gentle Mothering*, she quotes research from Dr. Diaz-Rossello, "All the evidence shows that the best bank for that blood is the baby."

Vaginal Birth and Gut Flora

The word *descendant* comes from the fact that our babies descend through the birth canal, which is important for baby's immune system. Baby's first inoculation is not breast milk or a vaccination, but descending through the birth canal. In a healthy normal person, billions of bacteria and microorganisms, called *microbiota* (or flora) reside in the gut, skin, and even in the vagina. When born vaginally, baby's mouth and nose are exposed to mother's vaginal microbiota. This beneficial flora from mother helps to seed and colonize baby's own intestinal tract with immune boosting microorganisms. Babies born by C-section are deprived of vaginal flora and lack a specific group of bacteria. According to a study from the *Canadian Medical Association Journal*, the birth—either vaginal or C-section—can influence a newborn's gut bacteria, and may have an impact on lifelong health. As research continues regarding the link between health and gut flora, children born by C-section have been shown to have higher rates of such illnesses as asthma, allergies, obesity, diabetes type 1, food allergies, and eczema. Vaginal birth is optimal because during pregnancy mother's birth canal changes to a higher concentration of lactobacillus which is the bacteria needed for milk digestion. In addition, research shows that babies born vaginally produce less gas and suffer less colic as a result.

Birth Wishes and Plan

There is the saying, "We plan and God laughs." However, keeping this in mind, you can still imagine the birth that you would like to experience. Some expectant couples write out elaborate birth plans of hopes, wants, and desires. Keep your birth plan simply written and concise. Be patient and know that life does not always go according to plan. Although we do not always know how we will respond, my birth teacher, Kathy, asked us to complete the following phrases:

- ✿ My top priorities for this birth are:
- ✿ The kind of room I feel safe in is:
- ✿ The following people will help me feel comfortable and empowered during my labor:
- ✿ The following items (food, music, pillows, candles, nightgown) will help me feel comfortable during my labor:
- ✿ If my labor is slower than I expected, the following things will help me stay busy:
- ✿ The following things will help me deal with pain in a natural way:
- ✿ When the baby is first placed on my stomach, the following things are important to me:

Tips on Having a Natural Undisturbed Birth

With information available in books, classes, and on the Internet, pregnant women are more savvy than in our parents' day. Nowadays, we want to partner with our healthcare provider and share in the responsibility for our healthcare, including our births. Consider the following tips for both women and their support team:

Practitioner: Thoughtfully choose your practitioner and birthplace. Ask about rates of interventions from induction, episiotomies, epidurals, and cesarean section. It is important that you feel comfortable with your practitioner and look forward to your visits.

Birth team: Surround yourself with people who respect your birth choices. If having a hospital birth, consider hiring a doula who is familiar with the birth experience and who can be your advocate in the hospital. A doula can offer support to dad too. The caregiver's role is important. Ensure the birth space allows for privacy, and that lights, smells, and sounds are minimized. Remove the clock. Allow her to rest during contractions. Avoid small talk and unnecessary questions. Food and drink are important. Follow her cues, but offer sips in between contractions. Remind her to urinate hourly.

Birthright: Remind yourself that giving birth is a normal rite of passage, a process done by all of our woman ancestors. Contractions come and go, and in between there is a break—most of the time. Your body is designed to give birth.

Comfort measures: Birth classes offer a plethora of information for comfort measures including use of the birth ball. In addition, many couples have found birthing techniques from breathing to hypnobirthing to be invaluable. Keep on moving, change position, and if possible, labor in the water. Spiral motions of the hips allow baby to navigate herself easier through the birth canal.

Consider your provider's suggestions: Remember it is okay to not agree to everything without explanation, especially if it feels counterintuitive (i.e. inducing without medical reason). Use the BRAIN acronym (see Chapter 2), and ask about the option of patiently waiting and not doing anything prematurely. Regarding medications, comfort measures and a doula are alternatives to anesthesia.

After Birth: Mother and baby should stay together, preferably skin to skin. Encourage breastfeeding after birth. Maintain a serene atmosphere, keeping lights, sounds, and commotion to a minimum. If baby needs to leave for urgent medical reasons, father or another family member should stay with the baby. Measurements of length and weight can wait.

Interventions: Policies and Procedures

The wonders of the twenty-first century have given us technological achievements that greatly facilitate our lives. In the field of obstetrical medicine, there have also been tremendous advances especially in the management of high-risk cases. However, success has led to excess, and nearly all hospital births are subject to use of various interventions used routinely on everyone, and no longer reserved for only high-risk conditions or emergencies. Many women choose the hospital birth plan, yet are interested in having a low-intervention experience. It is said that, "knowledge is power," and in knowing what exists in various birth settings, one can aid the process by preparing ahead of time.

Intravenous Fluid Infusions (IV Fluids)

Intravenous Fluid Infusion therapy is often routinely used in the hospital during labor. The rationale for using IV fluids is to correct severe dehydration (usually due to continuous vomiting), for an epidural, or for a cesarean section. If there is an emergency, the IV line is already in place and can be used for immediate access. Some hospital policies require that a woman not be allowed to eat or drink and she is given IV fluids instead. This is in case of extreme emergency situations that require general anesthesia and surgery, preferably on an "empty stomach." However, laboring women rarely require general anesthesia for emergencies.

There are drawbacks to having intravenous fluid routinely when there is no medical necessity. Having IV fluid therapy and its equipment (poles and stands) impedes a mother's ability to move and easily change position, both of which are important for labor. Additionally, intravenous fluids are not an ideal replacement for food and water. In some hospitals, laboring women are offered ice chips. Labor requires great energy and stamina for which a woman needs proper food and drink. According to Ina May Gaskin, "Some hospitals—usually those where midwives have been able to influence policy by presenting the best evidence—allow women to eat and drink at will during labor. No poor outcomes have been reported from this change in policy."

When the intravenous fluid is given it is usually in large quantities. Studies show that IV fluids can accumulate, and women can become over-hydrated. This may lead to respiratory distress and seizures in both the newborn and mother. It can also inflate babies' birth weight in utero, leading to increased weight loss in the first 24 hours after birth. Some mothers complain of generalized swelling upon leaving the hospital as well. For an epidural, patients are given a large amount of IV fluid (bolus) to prevent her blood pressure from dropping as a result of the epidural anesthesia. In addition, the excess fluid dilutes mother's blood, which can affect her own birth hormones that are specifically designed to facilitate her labor and delivery.

Consider choosing a healthcare provider who allows mother to eat and drink, saving the IV use only for when medically necessary. In traditional cultures, women intuitively ate and drank lightly during labor, as they pleased. The research supports that women should be free to eat and drink in labor, as mother knows best. If hospital policy requires IV access, consider requesting a simple hep-lock be used, in which an IV needle is inserted into the woman's vein, but without fluids. It is taped securely to her arm, and she is free to move about.

Vaginal Exams: How Far Along Am I?

During pregnancy, the cervix (the neck of the womb) resembles the tip of a beer bottle, with a long neck and small opening. As pregnancy progresses and baby descends into the pelvis in position for delivery, the cervix begins to soften and shorten until it is paper thin, this is known as *effacement*. By the time of delivery, the cervix has opened and dilated, transforming itself to the appearance of a wide mouthed pickle jar.

At the end of pregnancy, and especially during labor, everyone wants to know, "How many centimeters?" The gold standard for predicting how a woman's labor is progressing is through assessing the number of centimeters (cm) the cervix has dilated. Through vaginal exams, a woman's cervix is measured ranging from 0 to 10 cm, completely closed to fully dilated, as a result of uterine contractions. However, research shows that this method is not precise for many reasons.

A woman can be dilated at the end of pregnancy, and not have her baby for weeks. Vaginal exams, unto themselves, are considered an intervention, and can carry risks. In addition to being invasive and uncomfortable, especially during labor, reasons to minimize or avoid performing a vaginal exam at the end of pregnancy and during labor include increased risk of human error in calculations, increased risk of infection, and accidentally rupturing membranes (breaking the water), although some practitioners intentionally do the latter, believing it will initiate or speed up labor. Additionally, there is the nocebo effect in which a woman who is progressing well during labor learns she is "only" 4 cm and can become discouraged because of "lack of" progress. One can dilate from 4 cm to 10 cm in a very short time. Likewise, a woman who is 7 to 8 cm on exam, could have many more hours until birth. Practitioners also make mistakes. Accuracy for determining cervical diameter ranges between 48 and 56 percent. Research that compared vaginal exams done on women in labor against others done on models indicated that practitioners' abilities to measure dilation can vary. In the study done on models, the greatest variances occurred among beginning practitioners (residents).

According to childbirth experts, there are additional markers that are telling about the progress of labor, such as monitoring uterine contractions, checking baby's station, and observing mother's response, through vocalizations and emotional behavior.

Labor Station: Your Baby Positions Herself

During pregnancy your baby is floating in a sea of watery amniotic fluid. Closer to the due date, baby descends into the pelvis. Baby's position, also known as *station*, is considered a helpful measure. The station is checked in a vaginal exam, and is measured with plusses or minuses with regards to baby's location relative to the bony projections in the pelvis (ischial spines). A baby floating higher up in the pelvis, five centimeters above the ischial spines, is at a -5 station. At birth, baby's head is at +4 to +5 station. There are methods used among birth caregivers and doulas that provide additional insight and go beyond the standard vaginal exam. Doulas are trained to observe a woman during labor: from vocalizations, smells, discharges, and emotions. Not one method is exact, but all offer information when used together.

Purple Line

In addition, researchers have begun to acknowledge the existence of a red/purple line that arises from the anal margin extending between the buttocks. In a study of 48 women who began labor spontaneously, the purple line was found in 89 percent of the women. A correlation was found between the length of the line, the station of the baby's head, and cervical dilation. It is believed that the purple line is due to vasocongestion at the base of the sacrum.

Electronic Fetal Monitoring

Electronic fetal monitoring (EFM) is used routinely in the medical model to monitor baby during pregnancy and also during labor and delivery. EFM is an ultrasound device which keeps track of baby's heart rate and measures mother's contractions. It can be used intermittently or continuously. Baby's heart rate is considered a good indicator of how he is doing. EFM is used for high-risk pregnancies and deliveries, for conditions such as preeclampsia, diabetes, small baby, premature labor (before 37 weeks), unusual vaginal bleeding, high temperature, multiples (twins or more), obesity, water breaking for more than 24 hours, and medicated births (pitocin, and epidural). With two flat sensors placed on the abdomen, the monitor is held in place with an elastic belt strapped around mom's belly.

Risks: When used continuously, EFM exposes baby to ultrasound waves, sometimes for long periods of time (see "Ultrasound" on page 40). In addition to possible risks from ultrasound exposure, the information can lead to misinterpretation and over diagnosis, which obligates the staff to respond. EFM is used for the majority of hospital births, on both low- and high-risk mothers. According to researchers at the CDC, the use of EFM during labor and delivery offers few benefits for the majority of deliveries which are low risk, and does not improve birth outcomes. In addition, it is associated with increased rates of cesarean section due to lack of reliability, making it difficult even for highly trained health practitioners to accurately interpret. With EFM, mother is not allowed the freedom to move as she pleases, which is important for optimizing baby's heart rate and baby's position, and for labor to progress. If you require continuous monitoring, consider the telemetry wireless unit (found in some hospitals), which allows mother to move about within a certain range.

Alternatives to EFM are fetoscopes and Dopplers, both used intermittently. A fetoscope is a noninvasive special stethoscope that can be used after 20 weeks of pregnancy, and the Doppler is a handheld ultrasound device. Both require the presence and expertise of a professional. If there are any concerns regarding baby's heart rate and contractions, the mother can be given advice on how to improve the situation, such as changing positions to optimize blood flow.

In summary, EFM is globally used yet has limitations for low-risk pregnancies, leading to higher rates of interventions, including use of forceps, cesarean, pitocin, and epidural anesthesia. For women planning hospital births, consider asking the practitioner ahead of time if he or she will allow EFM 20 minutes on, and 40 minutes off. This allows for the freedom to move and also allows staff to monitor by EFM if necessary.

Your Due Date

Compared to other mammals, human babies are born more immature, dependent, and helpless. For this reason, the length of pregnancy is important to allow baby to be born full term with optimal maturation of the vital organs including the lungs, liver, and brain, the latter being the last major organ to develop. A full-term pregnancy is considered to be 40 weeks, with a range between the 37th and 42nd weeks. (I enjoyed my pregnancy so much that I did not mind that my son Etienne arrived 13 days past his due date. It gave me more time to nest and rest.)

The traditional method to calculate a due date is known as Naegele's Rule, which adds 280 days (9 months + 7 days) to the first day of the woman's last menstrual period (LMP). For this to be accurate, it requires the exact date of the LMP, a regular 28-day cycle, and conception on day 14. However, for many women their period is not regular, and many are not able to remember their LMP. There are other ways that are considered more accurate. For example, if a woman knows her day of conception, the estimated due date (EDD) can be calculated by adding 266 days (38 weeks) to the date. In the medical model of care, ultrasound measurements of the fetal biparietal diameter (BPD) in the second trimester are considered most trustworthy.

Yet with all this information, it does not mean baby will arrive on the date, nor is this a deadline. Ultimately, due date is meant to be an approximation where length of pregnancies can vary by as much as five weeks. Even when dates are accurate, up to 70percent of women deliver 10 days before or after their due date, leaving only 4 percent of women giving birth on their actual due date. Research shows shorter pregnancies occur in women less than age 20, women pregnant with baby girls, smokers, and those who have had prior pregnancies. Additional factors that influence gestation include weight, prenatal care, medical or placental conditions, stress, nutrition, ethnicity, and even moon phases. Dr. Anne Marie Jukic of the National Institute of Environmental Health Science concluded, "I think the best that can be said is that natural variability may be greater than we have previously thought, and if that is true, clinicians may want to keep that in mind when trying to decide whether to intervene on a pregnancy."

Knowing the approximate due date is important because every week in pregnancy is critical in the development of the baby. At 35 weeks a baby's brain weighs two-thirds of what it will weigh at 40 weeks. If dates are incorrect or based on a woman's LMP, there is a chance of underestimating the time in utero which has led to women being induced who were not truly overdue. A baby born before 37 weeks is considered premature or preterm. Especially with the variability of dates, inducing labor before a baby is ready to be born can be a cause of health concerns affecting baby's future including developmental delays. There are also sometimes instances where inducing labor is based not on medical reasons but on convenience for the doctor, patient, and/or hospital.

According to ACOG (American Congress of Obstetricians and Gynecologist), the normal range to give birth is 3 weeks before the due date or 2 weeks after, roughly between 38 and 42 weeks. The EDD is used as an approximation and helps guide practitioners in assessing mother and baby throughout the different trimesters. Approximately 28 percent of mothers deliver after 40 weeks, and 10 percent of infants deliver after 42 weeks. Beyond the due date, most obstetricians will recommend electronic fetal monitoring to check baby's well-being based on movements, heart rate, and amniotic fluid.

Amniotic Fluid Levels

Amniotic fluid is contained in a sac that surrounds the baby in the womb. It helps to maintain temperature, it offers protection and cushioning, and it aids baby with lung development and digestion. Sometimes the fluid level can be higher (polyhydramnios) or lower (oligohydramnios). A common cause of low fluid level is dehydration which may be corrected by drinking more fluids and resting. Additional causes of oligohydramnios include being overdue, placenta conditions, early leakage of membranes, hypertension, diabetes, and fetal abnormalities.

According to Dr. Sarah Buckley, "Low amniotic fluid levels does not, by itself, give an accurate assessment of fetal well-being, and [its discovery] has been shown to lead to over diagnosis of problems." As a result, this has been the cause of unnecessary induction in otherwise normal babies. The fluid is measured according to the amniotic fluid index (AFI) taken from ultrasound. There are several ways to evaluate pockets of amniotic fluids by ultrasound, and there have been instances of false positive results. Normal levels range from 8 to 25. Closer to delivery, as baby continues to grow; the pockets of fluid naturally decrease. Stress, fatigue, and dehydration can all lead to an AFI of less than 5. However, home care measures of rest, increasing fluids, and stress reduction have been shown to improve outcomes and avert the need for induction.

Overdue

Pregnancies that last beyond 42 weeks are considered *post-term*, and are more common in first-time mothers and women who have delivered post-term before. Most babies born past their due date are healthy. The rationale for inducing labor is that the rate of complications, although rare, can increase past 42 weeks. This means bigger baby, less amniotic fluid, increase in meconium aspiration, as well as higher chance of cesarean section. Both preterm and post-term births are associated with a higher rate of mortality compared to pregnancies delivered at term. All in all, researchers conclude that despite the increased risks, most neonatal problems can be prevented with careful management. In the case of a large baby, mother's body has been found to adapt and be able to accommodate a larger baby. Use of medication to induce labor has been shown to interfere with the natural changes during labor and can actually cause a rebound effect ending in a more difficult birth.

Inducing Labor

Talk to other mothers and it is not uncommon to hear that many were induced. For genuine medical reasons, inducing labor is determined when the benefits outweigh the risks rather than waiting for the body to naturally go into labor. This includes cases of severe maternal illnesses such as diabetes, hypertension, or cancer, or when a baby is not growing properly or has died in utero. In a meeting on Appropriate Technology for Birth, the World Health Organization recommended that, "No geographic region should have rates of induced labor over 10%." However, according to a survey by cultural anthropologist Robbie Davis-Floyd at the University of Texas at Austin, 81 percent of women who deliver in U.S. hospitals receive the medication, Pitocin, to start or speed up labor.

There are many reasons why doctors induce labor. For some medical practices it is their policy to not allow a woman to deliver much past her due date; another common reason is that they believe baby is too big or mother's hips are too small. In addition, with busy schedules, many women are induced out of convenience without regard to possible risks for mother and baby. Even then, ACOG recommends that women not be induced until 39 weeks when fetal lung maturity has been established. Labor can be induced with medications including the prostaglandins (e.g. Cervidil and Cytotec) and Pitocin or it can be done manually by breaking the water or stripping (sweeping) the membranes. Sweeping the membranes can stimulate production of natural prostaglandins. Performed by a practitioner who inserts two fingers inside the cervix, there carries the risk of accidentally breaking the waters. All of the methods used interfere with the body's natural physiology and hormonal system, which can set up mother for a cascade of interventions that do not take into account short-term and long-term concerns, and probably could be avoided if we wait. In a study of 7,800 first-time mothers in the United States, researchers concluded that women who were induced were twice as likely to need a C-section. (See Chapter 5 for information on natural approaches to inducing labor.)

However, if induction is deemed medically necessary, the first phase of inducing labor usually begins with medications such as prostaglandins to help soften and ripen the cervix and make it more favorable for induction. Consider beginning with Cervidil which is inserted into the vagina for 12 hours. When using Cervidil, there is no need for intravenous fluids. It is often used before Pitocin and may be enough on its own. Inducing labor is not without side effects, and risks include uterine hyperstimulation, fetal distress, postpartum hemorrhage, and upset stomach. Because artificially induced contractions are stronger and more frequent than the body's own, induction has also been linked to maternal deaths from amniotic fluid embolism.

Misoprostol (Cytotec®) is a prostaglandin, which is indicated in the treatment of ulcers, but is also used for labor induction and cervical ripening. A major side effect of Cytotec is hyperstimulation of the uterus, which impairs blood flow to the baby and may rupture the uterus. According to ACOG, misoprostol should not be used on women who have undergone a previous cesarean delivery. After dilation, methods to induce contractions are begun with Pitocin, nipple stimulation, or breaking of the waters.

Pitocin (Syntocinon®) is a medication used to augment and induce labor. It is chemically similar to mother's own birth hormone, oxytocin. Oxytocin is a neurohormone released during sexual orgasm (in both men and women), and is responsible for initiating birth. In addition, oxytocin plays an important role in breastfeeding and in the human emotional sphere, namely with maternal-infant bonding. In the pharmaceutical insert, Pitocin is specifically for induction of labor in patients with a medical indication: to stimulate or reinforce labor, as well as to produce contractions during the third stage (delivery of placenta), and to control postpartum bleeding. Its primary use is to start or speed up labor when deemed medically necessary such as when a mother has a severe condition of diabetes, hypertension, or when the baby is in distress. However, most often Pitocin is overused for nonmedical reasons such as an elective induction. This requires that a woman be lying down, with an IV, and monitored with EFM. Elective induction is not usually optimal as it signifies that labor has not started. Mother's body is not ready, her cervix may be closed shut, baby may not yet be in an ideal position, nor may its organs be mature and fully ready for birth.

Major differences between Pitocin and natural oxytocin (produced by the body) is the way in which they affect the body and the brain. When birth is allowed to progress naturally without medications, oxytocin is secreted causing contractions to occur intermittently and gradually build. On the other hand, Pitocin is administered in a continuous fashion through an intravenous line resulting in longer and stronger contractions that are difficult to manage, less efficient at dilating the cervix than oxytocin, and that can increase stress on baby by reducing blood flow and lowering baby's heart rate. Pitocin, which does not cross the blood-brain barrier, also interrupts the normal cascade of mother's birth hormones, which can affect maternal-infant bonding and is associated with poorer breastfeeding outcomes.

In a study from the *Journal of American Medical Association Pediatrics (JAMA)*, findings show a link between use of Pitocin during birth and likelihood of developing autism. There was a 35 percent greater likelihood of developing autism, particularly in boys. Used by most obstetricians, an analysis suggests that Pitocin is not as safe as was once thought. According to the American Congress of Obstetricians and Gynecologists (ACOG), a new study found that Pitocin use can have adverse effects on the newborn, resulting in poorer health assessment at birth (lower Apgar scores) and increased admissions to the neonatal intensive care unit (NICU). Being on Pitocin restricts a woman's ability to move because she requires an IV and continuous EFM monitoring. This approach sets up a cascade that can lead to further interventions such as epidural for pain management and increased chance of cesarean section.

According to Dr. Michel Odent, "Oxytocin is the hormone of love, and to give birth without releasing this complex cocktail of love chemicals disturbs the first contact between the mother and the baby. . . It is this hormone flood that enables a woman to fall in love with her newborn and forget the pain of birth."

Typically Pitocin is administered if labor has not begun by 42 weeks, although there are many obstetricians who will begin induction just after the due date. It is also used to start or speed up labor if a woman has a severe condition such as hypertension, if labor has not started following several hours of water breaking (membranes ruptured), or if labor has stalled. When Pitocin is used to jump-start labor, consider beginning with a low dose, allowing 30 minutes between dosing if possible. If the cervix has opened after 5–6 cm, consider asking the nurse to discontinue the Pitocin to evaluate mom's natural response. If contractions are too painful or frequent, the dosage can be turned down. As a practitioner, I appreciate the best of both worlds, and I know that on some occasions, albeit rare, there are times when Pitocin is medically necessary. (See Chapter 5 for information on natural approaches to inducing labor.)

Meconium Aspiration

Meconium lines baby's intestine during pregnancy, and is the dark, tarry, sticky stool passed initially by the newborn in the first few days of life. After a few days of breastfeeding, baby's stool turns into the characteristic mustard seed consistency. If a baby is in distress before birth, she may have a meconium bowel movement while still inside the womb. Complications, such as lung problems, could arise if baby breathes it in the lungs right at birth. Factors that increase stress on the baby include maternal conditions such as hypertension or diabetes, difficult delivery, aged placenta, and post-term babies. If baby is responsive and active with normal Apgar scores, no treatment may be necessary. Otherwise, symptomatic babies are evaluated and treated depending upon severity, usually with excellent prognosis. Finding the greenish-brown meconium stain in amniotic fluids (or when water breaks) does not necessarily mean that baby is in distress, as it is common to have a light meconium stain when going past due date. Most cases of aspiration occur with the thicker meconium. According to Ina May Gaskin, medical inductions during labor increase passage of meconium, most likely because the baby is more stressed than it would be if labor were left to begin on its own.

Pain Relief: History in Medicine and the Natural Birth Movement

Pain management options for childbirth in the medical world have developed significantly over the past century, but not without consequences. By the early 1900s, doctors were using 'Twilight Sleep," a combination of morphine and scopolamine which produces amnesia, causing women to forget their birth experience. In the 1920s and 1930s, a combination of opiates and barbiturates replaced twilight sleep. Due to being heavily medicated, women were unable to efficiently push during labor, which led to an increase in the use of forceps to pull baby out of the birth canal. It also led to an increase in cesarean section use. In addition, babies were born compromised and often required resuscitation for respiratory depression, and severe drug side effects contributed significantly to both mother and infant mortality.

After decades of medications that interfered with the birth process on physical, mental, and emotional levels, a new movement in favor of a more natural approach began to emerge by the 1930s. Early proponents of the natural childbirth movement favored nonmedical techniques such as breathing, hypnosis, relaxation methods, and water immersion. Popular teachings included Grantly Dick-Read (1943), Lamaze (1960), Leboyer (1975), and Bradley (1978). The publications of British obstetrician Grantly Dick-Read—*Natural Childbirth* (1933) and *Childbirth Without Fear* (1944)—expressed concerns about the use of obstetrical anesthesia, as well as the neglect of a woman's psyche during the experience. "Interference is still one of the greatest dangers with which both mother and child have to contend," he wrote. Fear of childbirth and the anticipation of pain leads to muscular tension in the body which closes the womb, known as fear-tension-pain syndrome. His ideology linked obstetrics with psychology, and ultimately focused on a belief system that childbirth without drugs could actually be an exalting, ecstatic experience. Different from popular thought of his day, he believed that childbirth was a woman's greatest honor and one of the most important events in a woman's life.

By the mid-twentieth century, "saddle blocks," a form of spinal anesthesia, became popular replacing the Twilight Sleep. Although the saddle block brought pain relief, women continued to have problems with pushing, which still often required the use of forceps. Refinements in spinal anesthesia have led to epidural anesthesia which is the most common method of pain relief for childbirth today.

Epidural Anesthesia

In industrialized countries approximately 50 to 70 percent of women will receive an epidural during labor. An epidural provides regional anesthesia by blocking the pain in the lower half of the body during labor and for cesarean section. With an epidural, the mother is alert, and the pain relief can also allow her to rest.

The epidural is given by an anesthesiologist (or nurse anesthetist) who inserts a needle in the area around the spinal cord in the lower back, leaving a catheter in its place. The medications used include narcotics such as fentanyl, in combination with anesthetics. Fentanyl, also used for cancer pain, is 50 to 100 times more potent than morphine. Although modern medicine claims epidurals to be the safest form of obstetrical anesthesia, it is not a benign procedure. Research on the side effects of epidurals on babies is somewhat ambiguous. According to the American Pregnancy Association, "Since dosages and medications can vary, concrete information from research is currently unavailable." Some of the known side effects for the baby lead to poor positioning in the birth canal, decreased heart rate, problems with breastfeeding because of trouble with latching, and breathing difficulties. All these consequences share an increased risk of a need for interventions such as forceps, vacuum, episiotomy, and cesarean section.

Epidurals affect each woman differently. Some women are paralyzed from the waist down during labor, while others are still able to feel the contractions, but no pain. Ten to fifteen percent of women will complain of inadequate pain relief, while one out of 20 women will not receive any pain relief from an epidural. Risk factors that increase the possibility of no relief include a woman who has given birth before, obesity, cervical dilation more than 7 cm, opiate users, and anyone with a history of previous failed epidural. According to Dr. Sarah Buckley, ". . . epidurals are associated with major disruptions to the processes of birth. These disruptions can interfere with a woman's ultimate enjoyment and satisfaction with her labor experience, and may also compromise the safety of birth for mother and baby."

However, in general many women are satisfied with the pain relief from an epidural. Epidurals require that a woman be lying in bed with continuous electronic fetal monitoring, with an IV drip in place. She may also have a urinary catheter. Although uncommon, there are a few hospitals that offer a newer anesthetic technique called a combined spinal epidural (CSE), known as a walking epidural, which allows a woman to move about.

Women can sometimes feel pressured into getting an epidural on the premise that the anesthesiologist is very busy, but able to take her at that moment. Side effects from the puncture include bleeding, headaches, and in some cases, permanent spinal damage. In an article in *Midwifery Today*, Judith Slome Cohain aptly points out that women who are able to sit still and quietly breathe through strong contractions during the 10 minute procedure for the epidural, probably possess the wherewithal to tolerate the rest of labor, without any medications. Receiving opiate pain medication through an epidural requires continuous monitoring with EFM because of the possibility of side effects on both mother and baby. All medications the mother receives cross the placenta and can affect her baby. According to one study, babies delivered with epidural use had lasting effects including higher rates of crying, fussiness, and less alert time in the first month following birth. Most women are not fully informed of the possible risks to both mother and baby.

There are cases where women have become permanently paralyzed, experience chronic headaches, and have even died from epidurals. The dynamics of birth completely changes with an epidural and can lead to failure to progress and ultimately to cesarean section. Sometimes the medication is discontinued to allow a woman to push during delivery, but the pain may return with a rebound effect of increased pain because the medication interferes with the body's own natural pain relief system.

Possible side effects from epidural anesthesia include the following:
- ❀ Decrease in maternal blood pressure which can lead to less oxygen for the baby.
- ❀ A slower, longer labor because mother is unable to stand up and move around, which contributes to less than optimal positioning of the baby in the birth canal.
- ❀ Maternal fever in labor. (When mother has a fever in labor this increases the likelihood that baby will be evaluated for possible infection and treated with antibiotics prophylactically.)

- ✿ Increased probability of need for neonatal monitoring and antibiotics.
- ✿ Increased risk of interventions such as forceps, vacuum extraction, and cesarean section.
- ✿ Difficulty with urination which may require use of a urinary catheter, which increases chances of a urinary tract infection.
- ✿ Leg paralysis and paraplegia (1 in 250,000).
- ✿ Itchy, red chest (also known as fentanyl itch).
- ✿ Backache at the site of the puncture wound, including chronic back pain.
- ✿ Migraines and headaches occurring during and after birth, sometimes lasting for weeks.
- ✿ Poorer birth satisfaction due to interference and lowering of mother's birth hormones, which affect delivery as well as the feelings of profound joy and ecstasy.
- ✿ Breastfeeding difficulties due to poor latching on by baby.

The aim of modern obstetrics and the use of epidurals is to ensure a positive birth experience through management of childbirth pain. There are women who are greatly aided by the respite from the pain and fatigue from the epidural, especially in prolonged labors. Because of the time for rest, some mothers believe they have had successful vaginal deliveries *because* of the epidural. With regards to pain medications, do not feel pressured. Labor and delivery nurses can be excellent; however, since they are assigned to several patients in the same shift, they have less time to spend with each patient, and often rely on medications to take the place of another human being. If the nurse offers medications and you are not interested at that moment, you can let her know you will ask if needed. It is better to make decisions when you are not feeling pressured. If you desire pain relief, and you originally wanted a natural birth, consider asking the nurse to return shortly. In the meantime, work with your coach to try different comfort measures such as changing your position, using a birth ball, pressure points, warm bath, cold washcloth, and so on. Sometimes making small changes brings great relief, which can allow you to better tolerate the contractions (see "Doulas" in Chapter 2).

Pregnant with twins, I accompanied my childhood friend, Mickie to the hospital for delivery. She was encouraged by her physician to get an epidural early on with induction of Pitocin. Completely numb from the waist down, she applied makeup with ease during "transition," a time in labor which is known for being one of the more difficult phases in labor. She marveled at this, and I had to admit, I was impressed too. However, an extremely difficult delivery ensued, and she was left with a high fever and nausea. She did not see one of her twins for over 24 hours, which also led to complications with breastfeeding. This reminded me that in life there are no "free rides." Childbirth is appropriately termed "labor" because it is meant to be hard work. When labor is complicated by medications and interventions, chances are the healing phase takes longer than a natural, undisturbed birth. See "Postpartum Wound Care" in Chapter 5.

Cesarean Section

Cesarean delivery, also known as a C-section, is used to deliver a newborn via an incision (cut) which is made in mother's belly and uterus. Cesarean delivery is considered major abdominal surgery, and in some countries, such as the United States, it is the most common surgery performed. C-section received the name from the common belief that Julius Caesar was born from a surgical birth. In the past, cesarean sections were performed only when mother was dead or dying, and there was a possibility to save the child's life. It was not until the 1800s, with improvements in medicine, that women had the possibility of surviving a cesarean section along with the baby. The rise of urbanization in the West that occurred from crowded living conditions in the city at the beginning of the twentieth century, witnessed an increased need for cesareans due to nutritional deficiencies such as rickets, which causes bone deformities, including of the pelvis, thus necessitating the cesarean section. With improved nutrition status and less pelvic deformities, the cesarean section rate should be lower. However, in 1970 the rate was approximately 5 percent, and it has since been on the upswing.

Currently, cesarean delivery rate in the U.S. is 30 percent for first-time mothers and 11 percent for women who had other children. The most common reason cited for cesarean section was failure to progress (35%) followed by abnormal fetal heart rates (27%), and poor positioning of the baby (18%). Of the patients who had a C-section for failure to progress, 40 percent were taken into surgery in early labor, with the cervix at less than 6 cm dilation (full dilation is 10 cm), and 30 percent of C-section deliveries occurred during the pushing phase of labor, at less than 3 hours of pushing. In other words, cesarean section appears to have been done too early and too soon in many cases. I feel this reveals a "failure to be patient."

Labor management by obstetricians is traditionally held to a standard called the "Friedman Curve," which guides the practitioner on parameters for a normal length and pace of labor. The Friedman Curve is a graph with defined guidelines for the average length of time for women to dilate in labor. If she does not dilate according to the plotted graph, then she may be given the diagnosis of "failure to progress." Published in 1955, the Friedman Curve is still used by most physicians to manage labor and delivery. However, current researchers believe that the Friedman Curve is outdated because birth practices, medications, as well as maternal considerations such as age and weight, are different today than they were nearly 60 years ago.

Home birth practices such as at The Farm Midwifery, where midwife Ina May Gaskin practices, have a C-section rate of 1.7 percent. In order to accomplish this low C-section rate, Gaskin and her partners emphasize an overall healthy approach including nutritious diet and exercise, and they work with women to reduce the fear and anxiety current in the West about birth, to help demystify the experience. For women who are given the option of an elective C-section, I urge you to make an informed decision, and consider the benefits both you and your baby can reap from a vaginal birth including boosting baby's immune system which can have an impact on health in later years (see "Vaginal Birth and Gut Flora").

However, there are times when a woman genuinely benefits from a C-section such as when there are problems with the placenta detaching or covering the opening of the cervix, which is the neck of the womb. However, one of the most common reasons cited for cesarean section is cephalo-pelvic dysproportion (CPD), which occurs when the baby's head is too big to pass through mother's pelvis. In Gaskin's experience, this situation of small hips and a large baby rarely necessitates a C-section in the midwifery model of care (see "Postpartum Wound Care" in Chapter 5).

Large Baby, Small Pelvis: The Myth about Cephalo-Pelvic Disproportion (CPD)

Cephalo-pelvic disproportion (CPD) occurs when baby's head is too large to pass through mom's pelvis. In past centuries, there were instances where CPD prevented vaginal births because of pelvic shape abnormalities caused by poor nutrition, rickets, and polio. Due to the reduction in infectious diseases and improvements in standard of living, including sanitation and nutrition, CPD is rare nowadays and may be due to congenital pelvic abnormalities or fractures causing a misshapen pelvis. Without proper diagnoses many doctors associate "failure to progress" with CPD. When in fact, it could be due to many factors including medications, positioning, or birth attitude on the part of both patient and doctor. CPD is difficult to diagnosis because it includes factors which are difficult to measure ahead of time. First, the ligaments in mother's pelvis soften allowing it to expand; this process is facilitated by the hormone, *relaxin*. Positions in labor such as squatting allow for 30 percent more pelvic capacity. The fetal position needs to be taken into account as well as baby's head which is comprised of moveable bones which can adjust to the size of the birth canal. All of these factors cannot be predicted ahead of time. However, it is common to hear a doctor tell a pregnant patient to expect problems with a vaginal delivery because her baby is too big for her pelvis. Comments like these only serve to increase anxieties (nocebo effect), and in some cases lead to self-fulfilling prophecies, ultimately resulting in cesarean section. Research has shown that women who previously had cesarean section due to "failure to progress," have been able to deliver subsequent babies vaginally, including larger infants than the previous one. In truth, women are designed to deliver babies vaginally... or our species would not have survived!

VBAC (Vaginal Birth after Cesarean)

One reason that led to increased C-section rate was the opinion that "once a cesarean section, always a cesarean section." Soaring healthcare costs combined with patient dissatisfaction led to the beginnings of vaginal-birth-after-cesarean groups (VBAC) such as ICAN (International Cesarean Awareness Network). Finally obstetricians responded and agreed to recommend as a standard of care a trial of labor in low-risk women who had previously had cesarean sections. According to the American Congress of Obstetricians and Gynecologists (ACOG), one of the contributing factors for the rise in C-sections from 5 percent in 1970 to 32.3 percent in 2008, was that there were fewer vaginal births after cesarean section (VBACs). Many hospital policies restricted doctors from a trial of labor after cesarean (TOLAC). By 2006, VBACs decreased to 8.3 percent. In 2010, ACOG issued new guidelines for obstetricians, "Attempting a VBAC is a safe and appropriate choice for most women who have had a prior cesarean delivery, including for some women who have had two previous cesareans." Obstetricians were urged by the ACOG President Richard N. Waldman, M.D. to "recommit to do everything in our power to reduce the cesarean rate." In nonemergency C-sections, the transverse incision, a horizontal bikini cut across the abdomen above the pubic area, is the current choice by most surgeons. It also allows the woman the option of having a VBAC for the next pregnancy. The classical vertical incision (from below the navel to the pubic area) may be used in emergency situations as it allows quicker access to the baby. With the vertical incision there is a higher chance of rupture of the uterus with future deliveries, and it is recommended to have a repeat C-section for the future.

But other reasons have contributed to the rapid rise in C-sections and these include technological, cultural, professional, and legal factors. According to the U.S. National Library of Medicine at the National Institutes of Health (NIH), "The growth in malpractice suits no doubt promoted surgical intervention, but there were many other influences at work." In the U.S., C-sections are a big moneymaker for both doctor and hospitals. With current insurance reimbursements, doctors are compensated less and have to work more. A woman's attitude about childbirth, her desire to have a vaginal birth, as well as the support of her birth team and healthcare provider, can all affect the outcome of the birth. Some mothers who have had a previous C-section elect to have another C-section based on the belief it is easier and more convenient. During a C-section, there are pediatricians in the operating room who evaluate the newborn because there can be more complications following a C-section than with a normal vaginal delivery. In the end, the child is deprived of experiencing the different stages of labor that are important for baby's health. Going through the birth canal squeezes the fluid out of the lungs at the time of birth. For this reason, babies born by C-section are more prone to breathing difficulties such as transient tachypnea of the newborn, abnormally fast breathing, and other types of respiratory distress.

Having a C-section often interferes with the normal birth experience which includes placing baby on mother's chest for breastfeeding. This can delay breastfeeding which may affect milk production. However, a woman's attitude towards breastfeeding plays an important role. According to Dr. William Sears, "Women whose babies are born by cesarean surgery are just as successful at breastfeeding as mothers who deliver vaginally as long as their commitment to breastfeeding remains high."

A C-section is major abdominal surgery and similar to other operations there is increased risk of bleeding, infection of the wound and uterus (endometritis), scar tissue, trauma to other organs, fertility issues, reaction to anesthesia, blood clots, and complications for the next pregnancy, including risk of uterine rupture and placenta complications. Because of the surgery, it also takes longer to recover from a C-section than a vaginal delivery. And like other types of major surgery, C-sections also carry a higher risk of complications. (See "Postpartum Wound Care" in Chapter 5.) Although most women do not intend on having a C-section, consider having a discussion with your obstetrician about his or her surgical technique. It is preferable that the uterus be closed in two layers of stitching, called double-layer uterine suturing, instead of a single layer. The double-layer is important in uterine scar healing and carries a lower rate of uterine rupture for subsequent labors, including a VBAC next time around.

Like many other medical interventions, success had led to excess. Reliance on high-tech features for pregnancy and childbirth do not come without a cost. The public dissatisfaction with soaring cesarean rates and other interventions have prompted natural birth organizations and coalitions to become more vocal about encouraging women and their practitioners to choose to have vaginal deliveries instead of unnecessary surgery. It is only recently that the idea of a fetus as a patient has begun to be of importance, largely due to sophisticated technology that makes it possible to visualize and monitor the baby in utero. Although there may be many complaints of the interventions employed in modern obstetrics, it is important to also note that the lives of many women and babies have been saved by avoiding such measures as cesarean section.

Episiotomy

An episiotomy is a surgical incision that is used to widen the vaginal opening during birth. The cut is made along the perineum, which is the soft tissue located between the vagina and the anus. In 2002, episiotomies were performed on 25 percent of all vaginal deliveries. Although it has been used routinely by many obstetricians who believe it prevents tears and facilitates a vaginal birth, ACOG has recently recommended against routine episiotomy and recommended that it should be restricted for emergency cases when it is vital to deliver baby immediately.

The reason for this recommendation is that once cut, the perineal tissue can more easily tear, than if it had not been cut at all. Such tears can lead to extensive 3rd- and 4th-degree tears with lasting effects. Approximately 40 to 85 percent of women will tear naturally, and two-thirds will require some stitches. Women who have had episiotomies, especially with extensive tearing, complain of slower recovery from birth and can suffer from painful sex and urinary and fecal incontinence. The incision can be either midline or mediolateral (a cut directed at a 45° angle from the midline.) A first-degree tear involves the skin, and may not need stitches. The standard episiotomy is a second-degree tear of the skin and muscle. Second-degree tears and more extensive ones require stitches (dissolvable) and the deeper the cut, the longer the recovery time. Complications are more common following the midline episiotomy, which is a straight cut from the vaginal opening to the anus.

Most women's birth plans include avoiding an unnecessary episiotomy. Women can prevent or minimize the need for an episiotomy by choosing an obstetrician or midwife who has a low episiotomy rate. During the actual delivery, practitioners can work with mother on such things as optimal pushing positions and delivery techniques such as use of lubricating oil, warm compresses, and gentle pressure on baby's head during crowning. Any modalities or intervention, such as electronic fetal monitoring, Pitocin or epidurals, which interfere with the natural birth process and limit mother's movement, position, and ability to optimally push, all can increase damage to the perineum.

In the journal *Midwifery Today*, Elizabeth Bruce ("Everything you Need to Know to Prevent Perineal Tearing") writes, "Avoiding epidural also helps prevent perineal damage. In one study, women with no anesthesia had the highest rate of intact perinea (34.1%), and women with epidurals had the highest episiotomy rate (65.2%). Another study shows that with an epidural women are more than three times as likely to suffer third- or fourth-degree tears."

Bruce also writes about the importance of position during labor. The semi-propped position, and the outdated flat-on-the-back lithotomy positions for pushing, which historically have been used in hospitals, are counterproductive for giving birth without the possibility of damaging the perineum. Birthing chairs and stools are better; however, being in a chair still limits ease of movement. A better position with minimal tearing would be the all-fours position, which offers maximum opening of the pelvis and relaxation of the perineum. In an ideal situation, with each contraction mother's movements will shift and adjust, and cannot be predicted nor orchestrated ahead of time.

Knowing this beforehand, I learned about preparations that I could do at home which might prevent or minimize tears. I attribute the ease of my deliveries (both boys were 8½ lbs), to the support and expertise of my midwife and birth team, as well as to my own preparation. Being able to participate in my upcoming delivery built my confidence, improved my attitude, and helped to demystify my body and the delivery itself. One of the things I did to prepare for delivery was perineal massage (see "Perineal Massage" on page 72 for more details). (See "Postpartum Wound Care" in Chapter 5.)

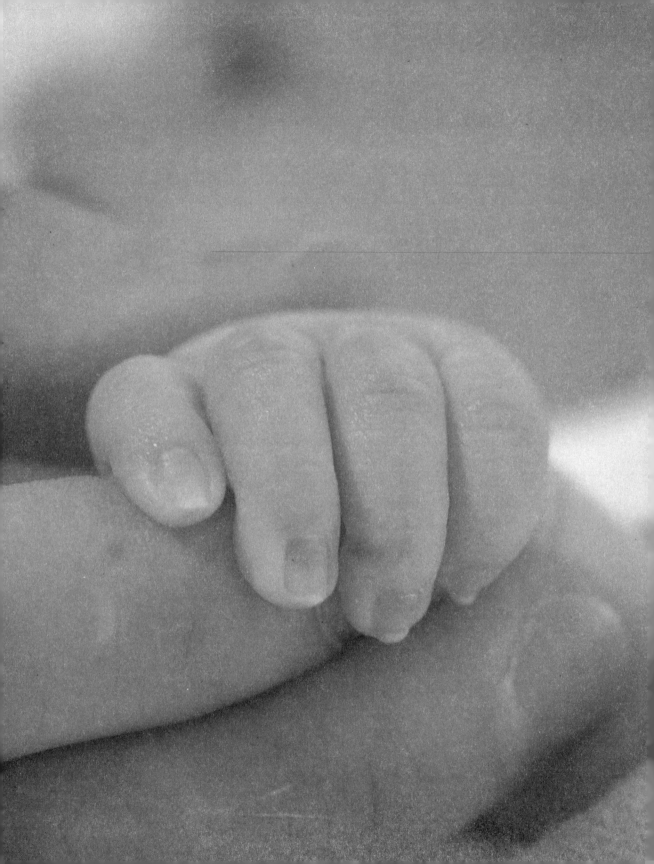

The Emotions of
Pregnancy and Birth

The Role of the Father

Go to any birth class, and it is common to see both expectant mothers and fathers in attendance. Most couples would not want it any other way. However, this has not always been the case. Over the centuries, childbirth has been a woman's business. Women were supported by other women during labor, with father only peripherally involved, if at all. It has only been in recent centuries, with the evolution of medicine, that male doctors have become interested in childbirth, particularly the medicalization of the experience (see "Introduction to Natural Pregnancy"). By the 1960s, fathers became included, and were expected to enter the delivery room arena—goodbye cigars! Interestingly, this parallels a time when hospitals became larger and less personal, and in the United States, midwives were less present. Hence, a familiar person, the father, emerges onto the childbirth scene.

My husband accompanied me to my birth class and participated in the exercises. When I went into labor with our first child, I woke him up in the wee hours of the morning. My contractions were climbing, and I really wanted him to press on my back, but he kept falling asleep, so I called my friend, Julie, who rushed over at 4:30 a.m. She stuck by my side until my son was born. This worked out best for everyone. I appreciated having my husband there, but I could see he was more comfortable boiling the water and doing other activities assigned to him by the midwife. Later on, I accompanied my friend, Susie, to the hospital for the birth of her second child, which consisted of only thirty minutes of hard labor. Although I thought she had a wonderful birth, I glanced over to her husband who was weeping in the corner, traumatized by the whole experience. He was there because he felt obligated to be with us. While sitting by my friend Karin's side while she was laboring in the bathtub, her husband came into the bathroom eating a bagel with cream cheese. He wanted to check in with her to see if we needed anything. Although he meant well, she was clearly irritated by the smell of the food and his conversation.

Most fathers have never witnessed a birth nor had any significant training besides a few childbirth classes, yet there are demands placed upon him that are beyond that of a medical student. Fathers are expected to act as coach, guide, and advocate without any professional training. As a woman's contractions intensify, most men become uncomfortable and can even become distressed in seeing their wife in pain. For a layperson this is a normal response. In addition, studies show that men and women tend to act differently toward the laboring woman. During labor, women touch a laboring woman more frequently, while men prefer to talk. Trying to converse with a woman in labor can interfere with the birth process, which is more about "letting go" to another consciousness, and less about engaging the intellect (known as neocortex activity). As a result, male partners are not always able to offer the type of support a laboring woman needs. The man's role in labor can be one of three possibilities: coach, teammate, or witness. The coach assists the woman during her contractions, while the teammate takes his instructions from the laboring woman or practitioner. The most common role is that of a witness who observes labor and is there to "hold the woman's hand."

After attending many births from my medical training to all of my close friends, I have come to realize that being at the birth is not fitting for everyone, including (in some cases) the expectant father. I have witnessed fathers who want to participate fully, and some who step back and allow others to help. There is no right or wrong way. Many fathers do not really know how they will respond until the birth day. Although there are wonderful stories of fathers who have been the ideal birth companion, this does not apply to all men. I have met quite a few men who confided in me that witnessing their wives birth was not a positive experience.

Research shows that male partners play a minor role in labor support, but it is still meaningful for most couples that he is present. In many cases, having her companion present during labor has a positive effect on a woman's satisfaction with the birth experience. Working with a professional, such as a doula, is a wonderful support for both the laboring woman and expectant father. In the end, if a woman desires a natural undisturbed birth in the hospital, I strongly recommend hiring a doula (see "Doulas" in Chapter 2).

Unexpected Results: What to Do with the Information

According to sociologist Barbara Katz Rothman, author of *Tentative Pregnancy*, when a woman is faced with difficult decisions following a negative test result from such procedures as amniocentesis, she can experience profound grief. Many parents do not thoroughly consider the implications of these tests and simply consent to them, believing they are routine. In my case, my husband and I did not want to have a medical printout of our babies, as we would not consider a termination. However, as they have been raised in the age of TV, computers, and video games, many people view pregnancy as just another aspect of life that has become part of the technical experience. Regarding ultrasound, feminist Germaine Greer commented, "We don't believe anything is real these days, until we see it on TV."

For many, pregnancy is considered tentative, or uncertain, until the results of the tests are confirmed. When an expectant couple receives news that their baby will have a disability or may have a birth defect which will lead to early death or lifelong challenges, there is enormous pressure from the medical community to terminate the baby's life, and do it as soon as possible. To receive the news of a prenatal diagnosis is devastating, shocking, and elicits many feelings. It is advisable to not make any rapid decisions, but instead to wait and avoid making choices under pressure. Sometimes screening tests have been inaccurate, and the follow-up diagnostic test is normal, or the data was misinterpreted. Consider a second opinion. There have been instances where women have aborted a baby who actually was normal. Take the time to do some research and learn about people with disabilities, as many handicapped people enjoy full lives. I have met families with a child with

Down syndrome who speak of the great love and joy their "angel" brings to the family. After all, there are many children who are born without any conditions but become disabled in childhood following a trauma, illness, or a vaccine reaction. All of this brings up many questions including, what to do if there is a problem, what support is available for handicapped children, and how you might feel about terminating a wanted pregnancy. When these questions arise, the womb no longer feels like a safe, secure place. From ultrasound to amniocentesis, babies are being poked and prodded. As we anxiously await for the results, what messages are we sending to our babies?

Parents faced with a prenatal diagnosis of a genetic syndrome or severe condition in their baby must make a difficult decision. Although many parents who receive a grave prenatal diagnosis choose to end the pregnancy, there can be lasting psychological effects following the loss of a baby whether from miscarriage or termination of a wanted pregnancy. According to Dr. Sarah Buckley, "there is no evidence that women who have chosen termination are, in the long term, psychologically better off than women whose babies have died at birth; in fact, there are suggestions that the opposite may be true in some cases." Most couples tend to grieve in private following a miscarriage, and this is especially true in cases of a termination. Because of the stigma of abortion, many feel isolated. Studies show there can be long-lasting consequences including marital conflict, guilt, anger, and depression, all of which can be heightened because the parents carry the burden of knowing they made the decision to terminate. In general, death is an uncomfortable topic, and well-meaning family and friends may minimize and underestimate the profound loss for an expectant couple. Following a miscarriage or termination, some couples are hesitant to try again, while others report subsequent pregnancies to be filled with fear, uncertainty, and lack of attachment to the new baby. There are many resources for grief support including psychotherapy, counseling, and local support groups. Begin with your doctor or midwife. The Internet also offers a plethora of information including listings of local groups. In addition, many couples have received assistance through holistic forms of healing such as homeopathy, acupuncture, and osteopathy.

Pregnancy, Birth, and Sexual Abuse

There are many factors in our lives that affect our fertility, pregnancy, and labor— one of these is our emotional well-being. All the events and experiences in our lives, joyous as well as challenging, have contributed in part to who we are in the present. Although it is common for all women to anticipate birth with a certain amount of trepidation or fear, this can be compounded when a woman has experienced sexual abuse, either recently or years before. In such cases, painful memories, both emotional and physical, may resurface during pregnancy and during birth. From homeopathy to therapy, there are many modalities that may aid healing wounds. Women who have experienced abuse are encouraged to discuss this with their practitioner ahead of time, as this may facilitate the birth experience for both patient and practitioner.

Birth Trauma and PTSD

The term post-traumatic stress disorder (PTSD) is usually used in connection with events such as war, rape, accidents, and natural disasters. PTSD occurs from either witnessing or experiencing a threat (actual or perceived) of harm, death, or injury to oneself or to another. In these cases, it is normal to experience a "fight-or-flight" reaction to a fearful or dangerous event. In the birth world, women have suffered from PTSD as a consequence of miscarriage, abortion, or traumatic delivery.

PTSD is complex, and is grouped into several main categories: reliving the event, avoidance, and feeling overly sensitive. Reliving the trauma with flashbacks can be triggered throughout the day and can include physical symptoms such as accelerated heart rate, sweating, and difficulty sleeping. With avoidance, the woman will avoid reminders as a way to compensate for the trauma. She may feel detached or emotionally numb, with strong feelings of guilt, anxiety, and sadness. As a result, there is a lack of interest in participating in previously enjoyable activities. For those who feel overly sensitive, a woman can be constantly on edge and easily startled, with angry outbursts. The physiological reaction stems from the activation of the adrenals which are responsible for the fight-or-flight response. This can keep her in a constant state of tension which may interfere with daily activities. These responses are normal for a short period of time following the experience, when they are known as an acute stress disorder (ASD). However, in some women and their spouses these feelings continue as an ongoing condition, which is referred to as PTSD. When it becomes chronic, family and friends are less compassionate, urging mother to "snap out of it." But just as with many conditions we are plagued with, one continues to suffer beyond one's control.

For many women, pregnancy and birth are the culmination of womanhood. Our magnificent bodies are perfectly designed for bringing new life into this world and nurturing our babies beyond the womb. When our pregnancies and birth do not go as intended, profound feelings can set in. In my practice, I welcome newborn families on a regular basis. In our first meeting when baby is just a few days old, we discuss mom's pregnancy and birth. I enjoy meeting all my new families and hearing about their birth experiences, ranging from home births to C-sections. In my experience, women who have had a normal natural birth, undisturbed without intervention, usually feel a sense of empowerment and deep satisfaction. On the other hand, it is common for many of my patients who receive unnecessary medical intervention to experience a great sense of birth dissatisfaction. They describe it as a loss, as if they were cheated from having a profound experience. According to the Birth Trauma Association (BTA) some women experience PTSD from events that would traumatize anyone, while others have birth trauma from occurrences that are not so sensational but focused on lack of control or dignity, or hostile attitudes. Because there is so much emphasis placed on the woman, it is also important to remember that fathers can feel helpless as well. Research from Oxford University reports that men can also experience PTSD and its symptoms following traumatic births; these include extreme blood loss and other complications resulting in life-threatening situations. Hospital staff is encouraged to also attend to the father when needed, although many of these complaints can arise well after the actual birth experience. Although some of the symptoms of postpartum depression (also known as postnatal depression) and PTSD overlap, the two illnesses are considered different.

The BTA's list of triggers for PTSD includes:
- ❀ Lengthy labor or short and very painful labor
- ❀ Induction
- ❀ Poor pain relief
- ❀ Feelings of loss of control

- High levels of medical intervention
- Traumatic or emergency deliveries, e.g., emergency caesarean section
- Impersonal treatment or problems with the staff attitudes
- Not being listened to
- Lack of information or explanation
- Lack of privacy and dignity
- Fear for baby's safety
- Stillbirth
- Birth of a damaged baby (a disability resulting from birth trauma)
- Baby's stay in Special Care Baby Unit (SCBU)/Neonatal Intensive Care Unit (NICU)
- Poor postnatal care
- Previous trauma (for example, in childhood, with a previous birth, or from domestic violence, see "VBAC" in Chapter 3)

Postpartum Depression (Postnatal Depression)

When I was expecting my first baby, I was led to believe that the greatest hurdle I would face was childbirth itself. After that initial obstacle, the hard work was over and my "bundle of joy" and I could live, I hoped, happily ever after. It was true that childbirth proved to be a profound experience, accompanied by feelings of indescribable elation as well as exhaustion. Like most mothers, I was simply glad that labor was finished so that I could hold my baby. But I found, as all parents do, that even the first moments of my child's life brought a number of challenges. From lack of sleep to sore nipples, it was downright difficult! During the first few weeks after my birth, there would be times when I would be overcome with waves of emotions that left as suddenly as they came. Studies show that 40 to 80 percent of women experience disturbances probably due to hormonal fluctuations leading to elation, tearfulness, and sadness. These "blues" can come the first week after delivery, and usually resolve within two weeks.

Compared to our ancestors, the modern family's postpartum period leaves the new parents practically alone, to fend for themselves. There are high expectations in the West to cope soon after birth. This does not take into account that many mothers also need to heal from the interventions of an episiotomy scar, abdominal surgery from a C-section, or medication side effects. In the past, family members and friends would have been present in the household to take care of the new family's needs, pampering the new mother with special foods, and giving her a chance to rest, bond, and breastfeed. New mothers were not expected to participate in daily activities for at least 40 days (see "Forty-Day Period" on page 115). Ina May Gaskin writes, "Is it any wonder then, that the postpartum depression is the most common post-birth complication in our society?" For some women, the "blues" can develop into a postpartum depression (PPD), occurring on a daily basis, interfering with daily activities. PPD is complex and may be difficult for the family and their practitioner to recognize because of the generalized complaints among many new mothers from lack of sleep and exhaustion. In addition, women may be hesitant to share their feelings, because of the high societal expectations for becoming a mother. The postpartum period may also trigger pre-existing conditions such as anxiety, obsessive-compulsive disorders, and depression. Many of these symptoms go underreported because women feel ashamed to reveal that they have feelings of anger and resentment toward the baby. In the medical model, emphasis is placed on prescribing medication, rather than an at-home support team that can include family, friends, and also professional caregivers such as a doula.

Support and Treatment

When a woman suffers from a difficult event surrounding her fertility, pregnancy, or birth, feelings of grief are a normal response. Following a grieving period which varies between people, if complaints continue and interfere with daily activities and relationships, these are not a sign of weakness, but rather, an indication that it is a time to look for extra support and help. In the Western world, our lives are more solitary than they were in past generations. As a result, there is less support, and more isolation. To fill the gap, there are also more professional services available than ever before. If conditions are ongoing, it is important to seek professional help, including holistic treatment with a homeopath. Many women have experienced profound healing from past traumas, including PTSD. (See "Anxiety" and "Grief and Sorrow" in Chapter 5.)

Birth Spacing and Birth Control

According to Dr. Weston A. Price (see Chapter 1), primitive societies deliberately spaced their children approximately every two to three years because it was more optimal physically for the mother. It allowed her to recover her nutritional stores and her energy, and also gave adequate bonding time between mother, father, and child. Although a full-time breastfeeding new mom usually will not get her period for months, it is still possible to get pregnant. For this reason, your practitioner will discuss birth control options at the six-week postpartum visit.

Contraceptive Hormones

The oral contraceptive pill (OCP) is composed of a combination of the female hormones estrogen and progestin, or for breastfeeding mothers, the mini-pill which contains only progestin. In addition to the daily pill prescription, there are other hormonal choices such as the patch, vaginal ring, and periodic injections. All of these interfere with a woman's normal cycle, and are meant to prevent pregnancy. OCPs work by stopping the woman's ovary from releasing an egg during ovulation, and also cause thickening of the cervical mucus, making it difficult for the sperm to join the egg. This does not always happen and the sperm may still fertilize the egg, resulting in conception. In this case, OCPs also cause thinning of the uterine lining which would make it difficult for a fertilized egg to implant and thrive. With the standard prescription, women will have a monthly period; however there are other variations that extend the cycle to quarterly bleeding or no bleeding altogether.

Most practitioners and patients believe the hormonal method is harmless, and carries minimal to no risk, and in some cases is beneficial. Minor side effects of OCPs include weight gain, nausea, swollen breasts, spotting, and mood changes. More serious adverse reactions include gallbladder and liver disease, stroke, blood clots, hypertension, and heart disease. In addition, studies suggest that OCPs may increase the risk of breast cancer and can delay fertility (short term).

IUD

The IUD is a foreign body used to prevent pregnancy. This plastic device is placed into the uterus, attached to a string that comes out of the cervix and hangs into the vaginal canal. Two devices currently offered are the copper IUD (ParaGard®) which releases copper, known to be toxic to sperm, and the hormonal IUD (Mirena®) which releases progestin. IUDs affect the uterine lining by preventing implantation of a fertilized egg. In addition, both types of IUDs can damage and kill sperm. Common complaints related to IUDs include irregular bleeding and cramping. In a report by the FDA Adverse Event Reporting System (FAERS) there have been many cases of device dislocation of the hormonal IUD (Mirena), in which the IUD became embedded in the uterine wall, or had migrated out of the uterus altogether. Some women required surgery for perforation of the uterus. After witnessing a patient go through a miscarriage with the ParaGard® IUD in place, I decided to learn more. In my research, some studies confirmed what occurred with my patient; that a woman can still get pregnant because the sperm was able to fertilize the egg. However the IUD prevented the fertilized egg from implanting on the uterine wall, thus leading to miscarriage, complete with all the hormonal changes. Following this difficult experience, we no longer offer the IUD at our office.

Fertility Awareness Methods (For Preventing or Achieving Pregnancy)

There are several natural methods of preventing pregnancy known as fertility awareness-based methods (FA) and include the Billings Method, natural family planning (NFP), and Symptothermal. These methods are based on a woman keeping track of her monthly cycle and peak fertile times by charting her temperature, cervical mucus, and cervix changes—depending upon the method used. FA is considered highly effective as long as the guidelines are followed. It is appealing for couples because it is inexpensive, easy to use, and has no medicine side effects. Once the method is learned either from a book or an instructor, it is easy to chart and takes only a few minutes per day. In addition, couples can use these natural methods to achieve pregnancy as a woman becomes more familiar with her cycle and time of ovulation. Women who have not begun their period because of breast-feeding can also use this method.

As a physician who strives for a "best of both worlds" approach, my aim is to meet the needs of my patients in a way that is as natural as possible. I prefer to rely on natural methods and remedies that are safe and nontoxic, while prescribing standard medicine only when medically indicated. As with any medication or drug, OCPs and IUDs carry side effects, including miscarriage, and women should become informed before they consent to taking them. In addition, the use of hormones interfere with the natural rhythms of the body. For these reasons, my preference is for the use of fertility awareness methods.

Forty-Day Period

The first month after birth is characterized by intense intimacy between you and your baby, and will build the foundation for a strong bond throughout her infancy, childhood, and beyond. At this stage, she is dependent on you for everything—food, shelter, frequent changing, warmth, and love—and by meeting these needs you establish crucial trust and stability early in her life. This first month is part of the forty-day period in which it is recommended that mother and baby spend time together breastfeeding, resting, and bonding. When I was a child, our neighbor Connie spent several weeks resting around the house following the birth of her children. I was perplexed, since that kind of extended recuperation seemed old-fashioned. It was not until my own pregnancy that I learned about the age-old custom of the forty days, which I ended up adopting just like our neighbor and millions of women around the world. If there are other children in the family, this period will encompass family adjustments to the new baby. It is said that baby and mom should stay within nine feet of each other during this period. Although it is customary in our culture for friends and family to inundate you with social visits, resist these visitations and the obligation to entertain for several weeks. After all, what's the rush? You will always have the opportunity to introduce your baby to the world, but these first weeks together are irretrievable. The forty-day period can also help ease the transition into parenthood, which can be fraught with overwhelming and often conflicting emotions. During this time, it is important to protect your baby from too much stimulation and to allow mother and family to rest. A good rule of thumb is to sleep when your baby sleeps. Ideally, have friends or caregivers take care of all other activities, such as food preparation, errands, household chores, and helping with other children. In my own experience, giving my baby and myself a concentrated period of time together restored my energy, which I needed as I knew I would be going to work soon after. In fact, I have found that women who deny themselves this special period of rest and attachment can end up fatigued for several years. Do the best you can, ask for help when you need it, and be careful not to overdo it!

Everyday Tips for the Attached Parenting Marriage

FROM THE DOCTOR'S DESK

Connie and Tony came to the office for their 9-month-old son's check-up. Nicholas was fussy from teething, but otherwise was doing well and meeting his milestones. The parents spoke of being exhausted from frequent waking which had strained their once harmonious relationship. We spoke about ways to improve the situation, and the parents were given a "prescription" to go on a date once a month, just the two of them.

Your relationship as a couple is important for you, and for your children. Nowadays, many families embrace the model of Attachment Parenting (AP) which focuses on forming strong healthy connections and bonds between parents and their children. In honoring our children's emotional and physical needs, parents help build a foundation for a lifetime. However, sometimes, in trying to be devoted parents, the parent-to-parent bond and connection becomes neglected.

According to AP, parents are encouraged "to treat their children with kindness, respect and dignity, and to model their interactions with them the way we'd like them to interact with others." Unfortunately, while attending to daily activities, many couples struggle with finding time to consider one another's thoughts and feelings. It is a common tendency to take each other for granted. As a child's first role models are usually the parents, it is important that the parent relationship also display acts of kindness, respect, and dignity for one another.

There are many joys that come with a new baby. Everyone's emotions run high as life adjusts to breastfeeding, bonding, and lack of sleep and sex. Once baby comes, the relationship is now forever changed. Naturally an infant requires love and attention, but after the excitement settles, many parents are left in a state of confusion as their roles and relationship become re-defined, again and again.

From reading the latest research to attending classes, expectant couples spend many hours preparing for birth and baby. It seems that we prepare more for our newborns, than for our relationship, which is meant to last a lifetime. Compared to the past when young parents had support from family along with deep-rooted customs and traditions, many contemporary couples take their vows without any preparation or guidance. Nowadays when difficulties arise, we possess few resources, so it is not surprising that the divorce rate is nearly 50 percent.

When baby is born, couples may encounter new challenges regarding finances, religion, household chores, raising children, gender roles, and family values. Although there may have been discussions beforehand, a couple may not really know how he or she may respond until becoming a parent.

Attachment Parenting and child-rearing philosophies help guide parents and offer resources for the well-being of our children, as well as for the whole family. They are meant to be adapted to meet the family's needs. One of the important lessons we can learn from our children is that many things in life do not go as originally planned. It is important that parents remain flexible, strive for balance, and enjoy the experience. Ultimately, children learn by modeling their parents for nearly everything. According to the ancient proverb, "Give your children two things: roots and wings." Being a parent is an immense responsibility, yet it is extremely rewarding to participate in building a foundation for the next generation with the aim of raising children who act with kindness, respect, and dignity for themselves and others. For this reason, your relationship as a couple is important for you, but also for your children.

Everyday Tips for a Healthy Marriage

1. Communication. Slow to anger, quick to listen. Listen more than you speak. Consider the 95/5 rule: offer positive comments 95 percent of the time and constructive criticism 5 percent. As human beings, our tendency is to point the finger and blame others, especially our spouse. We often have unrealistic expectations of how our spouse should or shouldn't make us feel on a daily basis.

2. Consideration. Charity begins at home. In his book, *The Good Life: What Makes a Life Worth Living*, psychologist Hugh MacKay answers that a life worth living is a life lived for others. "The 'good life' is not measured by wealth, status, career success and levels of happiness, but is defined by our capacity for selflessness, the quality of our relationships and our willingness to connect with others in a useful way." This concept is based on a fundamental principle found in many faiths which states that we should treat other people the way we would like to be treated. Consider your spouse, and pay attention to his or her needs.

3. Intimacy. To have and to hold. Men and women are "wired" differently in many ways, including their hormones. As a result of adjustments such as lack of sleep and breastfeeding, for many couples (and especially for women), sex no longer takes precedence in the postpartum period. However, after baby is several months old, it is important for both parents to compromise. Remember, sexual intimacy helps to unite you as a couple.

4. Courtship. Rekindle your relationship. Go on dates on a regular basis (i.e., once a month). Consider a marriage retreat, or a weekend getaway. Share babysitting duties with like-minded families. If you are short on funds, skip dinner or a movie and go on a daytime hike.

5. Compromise. Set realistic expectations, and remain flexible.

6. Take care of yourself. Take an exercise class, or go on a walk or hike. For inspiration, set aside a minimum of 10 minutes each day (even up to an hour) for prayer, meditation, or reflection. When you feel good, it helps to recharge, refuel, and rejuvenate all aspects of your life, including your relationships.

7. Don't overextend yourself. Learn to say no. For some people, it is difficult to say no. As a result, this can lead to making commitments that are above and beyond the call of duty as a parent and spouse. For example, if life is extremely hectic, it may be best to not overextend with volunteering at school. Of course, marriage and parenthood are full of obligations, but it is best to choose your commitments wisely.

8. Ask for help. If difficulties persist, seek help with friends and family. Many couples have had success "working-it-out" with a therapist, minister, or other professional.

9. Homeopathy in the postpartum period (and beyond). Holistic medicine can strengthen a mother or father's constitution and address complaints such as mood swings, libido, and fatigue, all of which can affect our relationships. Following a nine-month pregnancy, birth, and breastfeeding, it is usually mom who is most physically affected. Due to the dramatic changes in hormones and lifestyle, along with lack of sleep, there are many remedy choices for her, and the whole family. (See "Anxiety" and "Grief and Sorrow" in Chapter 5.)

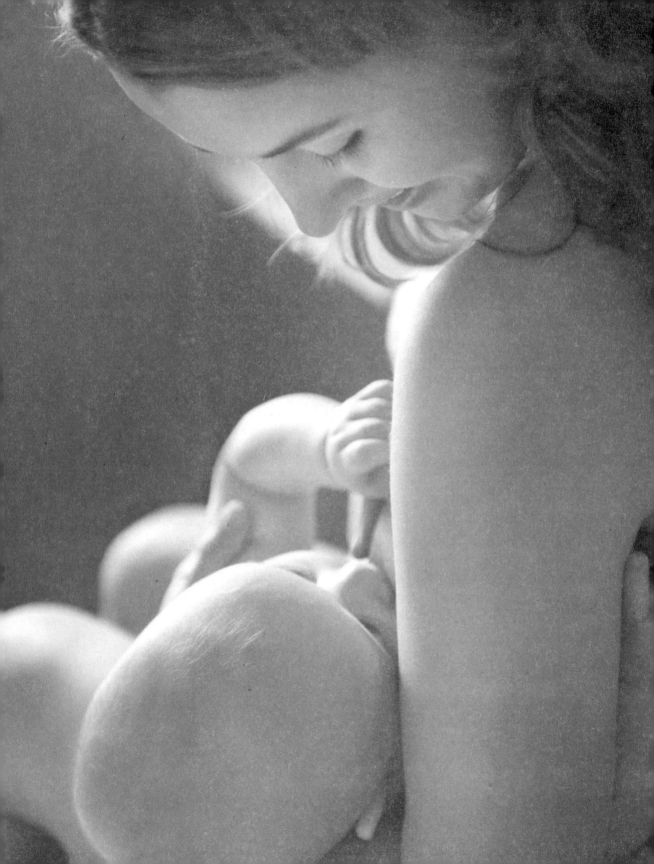

Natural Treatments and Homeopathy for Pregnancy Conditions and Childbirth

I N THIS SECTION, YOU will find a list of common pregnancy conditions, from hemorrhoids to nervousness. The homeopathic and natural treatment options given are for mild self-limiting conditions that usually do not require a practitioner's attention or prescription. Most of the entries describe conventional treatments for the condition, and give some suggestions for homeopathic and other natural remedies that may work either as alternatives or complements to the standard treatment.

Using Homeopathic Medicines
(also see "Introduction to Natural Pregnancy")

Homeopathy is a safe and gentle holistic medical approach, and most homeopathic medicines can be used in pregnancy. Homeopathic remedies are made from various plant, mineral, and animal substances. There are hundreds of homeopathic medicines for pregnancy-related conditions. Most are over-the-counter (OTC) medicines and few are available by prescription.

Homeopathic medicines (also referred to as remedies) are prepared through a series of dilutions and succussions (vigorous shaking of the diluted substance which activates the homeopathic medicine). In the preparation process, natural substances are diluted to the point where all that is left in the medicine is the "print" or the essence of the substance. Just as if one were to touch a pane of glass with a finger, a print would be left, though the finger would not be there. So in homeopathy, the energy of the substance remains in the remedy while any possible toxicity of the substance is diluted out. Such a process renders natural products nontoxic while increasing their potency, producing a safe and effective treatment.

Dosage

Homeopathic medicines for home use are available at health food stores, homeopathic pharmacies, or online. They are prepared by homeopathic pharmaceutical companies in a variety of potencies from 6 (6X or 6C) to 30 (30X or 30C) to 200 and higher; 30C is my preference, as it is easy to find in the stores. Counter to the intellectual thought process, a homeopathic remedy that is more diluted is considered stronger. Hence, *Arnica* 200C is stronger than *Arnica* 30C; the former is diluted 200 times compared to 30 times. In the end, the correct choice of remedy will work at any strength. In general, remedies in the strengths of 30C need to be repeated more often than those of 200C. Most homeopathic medicines are available in pellet form, which are round and spheroid shaped. In some instances, they come as tablets and this is dependent upon the manufacturer. They all taste sweet, and for this reason are child-friendly.

Directions for Use

Especially in labor, remedies can be taken in the 30C or 200C potency. Take 3 pellets up to three times per day under the tongue. In acute cases such as labor, a remedy can be taken every 30 minutes until there is relief, or as directed by your practitioner. If you see no improvement after three doses, discontinue the remedy. If a remedy needs to be taken often (such as *Arnica* 200C in labor), the remedy can be placed in water. Place three pellets in a glass of water and let stand for five minutes. Stir ten times. If you are using the hard pellets, they will not dissolve immediately, but the water becomes medicated. A teaspoon of the medicated liquid equals one dose. Avoid eating or drinking 10 minutes before and after taking the remedy. When possible avoid touching the medicine.

Substances to Avoid: During the time period that you are taking a remedy, it is best to avoid coffee, chocolate, camphor, eucalyptus, mint, and other strong-smelling substances (mint toothpaste is okay).

Persistent or Worsening Symptoms: If symptoms persist more than three days, or worsen, discontinue the remedy and consult your practitioner.

Improving Symptoms: As your condition improves, take your homeopathic medicine less often (one to two times per day). When you are substantially better, discontinue the medicine.

Storing and Traveling: Store your homeopathic medicines away from electrical appliances, strong-smelling substances, and extremes of temperature. If possible, have your medicines hand-checked at the airport, instead of going through the x-ray machine.

A Note on Chronic and Severe Illnesses

The homeopathic treatment of severe illnesses or chronic ongoing diseases like recurrent genital herpes, preeclampsia, and severe depression require the expertise of a professional, and are beyond the scope of this book. There are many conditions that are amenable to homeopathic treatment but require a more in-depth approach. In the classical homeopathic approach, the practitioner will spend approximately 1½ to 2 hours for the first visit with a child or adult. During this comprehensive interview, the practitioner is interested in gathering many details about your current condition, medical complaints, past history, lifestyle, mental and emotional attitudes, past traumas, character, and other relevant information.

Dr. Samuel Hahnemann, the father of homeopathy, wrote, "A single symptom is no more the whole disease than the single foot is of a man." A homeopath's goal is to choose a homeopathic medicine that matches the person's totality of symptoms, not just the main diagnosis. In other words, if five patients come to my office with complaints of infertility, each might be treated with a different homeopathic remedy because each person is an individual. With several thousand homeopathic medicines available, a properly chosen remedy that closely matches the individual can stimulate the body to begin to heal itself, strengthen the constitution, and address any ongoing conditions. In the case of a woman with complaints of infertility, this can optimize her potential to conceive and have a normal pregnancy. In this way, one medicine is used at a time, as constitutional treatment can have a profound effect on physical, mental, and emotional levels.

Case Taking

Similar to my book *Natural Baby and Childcare,* the following information offers a way to assess a complaint logically, and take appropriate action. In this way, one can remain composed during a stressful time. This information will also help your practitioner if you need to call on one. I am reminded of the quote by Teresa of Avila who wrote, "To worry over our health will not increase our health. This I know." People have commented to me that the ability to use homeopathy and natural medicines at home and offer themselves (or their family members) relief was very satisfying compared to the alternative of waiting and worrying.

In order to prescribe the correct treatment, consider "taking the case." Homeopathy and other forms of natural medicine expand your options for treating common ailments at home. In order to prescribe the correct treatment, however, you will need to begin to think a bit like a homeopath, going through the "case-taking" process that will lead you to choose a course of action or remedy.

Charting

To find the correct course of treatment, you must first compile a detailed history, which in this case could be yourself. I recommend you keep a journal, similar to the file your doctor has at the office. Having a *home chart* allows you to keep track of your observations and prescriptions. In medical school, we were taught a simple note-taking method that most practitioners still use in their practice known by the acronym, *S.O.A.P* (subjective, objective, assessment, plan). The *SOAP* note allows you to process your observations in an organized manner, and enables you to construct your home journal so that it keeps track of the same basic information. Keep the journal so you can use it for your baby soon.

Subjective

Under this heading you will write down the history of the complaint. As a *home practitioner*, you will want to make accurate observations about the condition, paying particular attention to the signs and symptoms that present themselves spontaneously and unprompted. If you are charting for a pregnant (or laboring) woman, avoid leading questions such as, "Does your back hurt?" This can often elicit a one-word reply just to placate you, so be sure to base your assessment on other factors, including observation. During labor, most questions and everyday conversation should be avoided anyway.

Symptoms

Symptoms are subjective sensations experienced by the woman herself, such as stomachache, headache, or nausea. They may not be apparent to others. Use the following questions to organize the "Subjective" section of your journal:

- ✿ When? Date each entry.
- ✿ What? List the main complaints. Begin with the most important ones first.
- ✿ Why? If you can pinpoint it, write down the cause.
- ✿ How? Indicate how this illness affects you (or her) mentally, emotionally, and physically. Include details particular to complaints, such as:
  - ✿ season (e.g., spring)
  - ✿ weather (e.g., damp)
  - ✿ time of day or night (e.g., 4 to 6 P.M.)
  - ✿ temperature (e.g., chilliness)
  - ✿ company (e.g., desires to be alone or clingy)
  - ✿ appetite (e.g., food cravings or aversions)
  - ✿ what makes symptoms feel better or worse (e.g., noise, light, touch)

Objective

The "Objective" section of the journal records the signs that others can observe such as irritability, redness of the cheeks, or restlessness. Examples include:

- ✿ Temperature (including thermometer readings)
- ✿ Energy level (e.g., exhausted or listless)
- ✿ Doubled over in pain

Assessment

In this section, you write your opinion of the problem. For your home chart, you do not need a formal diagnosis. For example:

- ✿ Morning Sickness
- ✿ Constipation
- ✿ Labor contractions, painful, early in labor

Plan

Here you write the treatment plan. It can be a remedy, home treatment, practitioner visit, or even a wait-and-see. For example:

- ✿ Sepia 30C
- ✿ Hot ginger tea
- ✿ Call the midwife, if not improved

Examples of Record Keeping

Let's look at two examples: Olivia, 28-years-old, pregnant for the first time; and Jackie, 37 years old, pregnant, mother of two. Both suffer from morning sickness in the first trimester. When you are determining a remedy, you will want to take into account both the objective and subjective aspects of the illness. One of the keys to finding the right remedy is to note every aspect that helps you to distinguish the condition, from the time of day the symptoms occur to the possible causes, to temperature readings and mood swings. Once you have taken down the full spectrum of the signs and symptoms, review the A to Z Guide which will provide you with a number of choices for remedies, varying according to the subtle differences among conditions. I have tried to simplify your search by providing several commonly used remedies for each condition, listing them with the symptoms they best treat.

Name: Olivia **Date:** Oct 23 **Age:** 28 years old **Notes:** In law school, and going through midterms	
SUBJECTIVE:	For the past several weeks, complains of morning sickness. Nausea all the time, especially in morning and after eating. Tendency to overeat. Sensitive to noise and odors. She is sedentary and is overworking while in mid-terms at law school.
OBJECTIVE:	Burping, vomiting, constipation, impatient, and angry with others.
ASSESSMENT:	Morning sickness.
PLAN:	Eat healthy, in small quantities, frequently. Rest, light exercise. Hot ginger tea. Nux vomica 30C—chosen as it is a good digestive medicine for heartburn and constipation associated with angry impatient mood, especially for people who are hard working. Called practitioner to inform him. Will visit him if the above measures do not help.

Name: Jackie **Date:** July 27 **Age:** 37 years old **Notes:** Stay-at-home mother	
SUBJECTIVE:	For the past several weeks, complaints of morning sickness. Constant nausea, especially in morning and late afternoon. Worse from smell of food. Craves sour foods that "cut" through the nausea. Has been irritable with children and husband, "I just want to be alone."
OBJECTIVE:	Easily irritated. Exhausted, wants to sleep. Feels better going to the gym at mid-day.
ASSESSMENT:	Morning sickness.
PLAN:	Rest, light exercise. Hot ginger tea. Sepia 30C—chosen as it is a helpful morning sickness medicine associated with feeling easily irritated and wanting to get away from it all. Called practitioner who said it was common at this time. Will visit her if the above measures do not help.

A to Z Guide to Pregnancy Conditions

ACID REFLUX

See *Heartburn*

AMNIOCENTESIS

See *Wound Care*

ANEMIA (IRON DEFICIENCY ANEMIA)

Pregnancy-related anemia is considered a common finding due to the physiological changes that occur to meet the demands of pregnancy. A pregnant woman's blood volume increases up to 30 to 40 percent, causing a temporary blood dilution, leading to a relative iron deficiency. Iron is a major component of hemoglobin (red blood cells) which carries oxygen throughout the body. According to Dr. Richard Moskowitz, "The diagnosis of anemia in pregnancy is probably not justified unless the hematocrit reaches 32 or lower with symptoms of fatigue, shortness of breath or palpitations." Iron deficiency anemia also causes chilliness, poor concentration, brittle fingernails, and frequent illnesses. It can lead to cravings for nonfood items such as clay, sand, and ice, known as pica. Dr. Michel Odent cites a large study which found the highest average birth weights were found in pregnant women who had a low hemoglobin (8.5 to 9.5) count while women with higher hemoglobin (above 10.5) had increased risk of low birth weight and preterm delivery. In other words, the studies did not necessarily demonstrate that iron supplementation improved birth outcomes. Despite this information, it is still advisable to ensure adequate intake of iron, preferably from natural sources.

Care and Treatment

Conventional Treatment

In addition to eating healthy, the standard medical approach is to prescribe an iron supplement (ferrous sulfate), however it can be poorly absorbed and causes constipation, heartburn, abdominal pain, nausea, and (less commonly) diarrhea.

Prevention and Home Treatment

- ✿ Encourage healthy eating including foods high in iron (see "Brewer Pregnancy Diet" and "Weston A. Price" in Chapter 1) such as dark leafy vegetables, watercress, seaweed, kale, beets, lentils, split peas, navy beans, white beans, kidney beans, garbanzo beans, firm tofu, tahini, whole grains, oatmeal, molasses, dried apricot, prune juice, raisins, pumpkin seeds, almonds, avocado, meat (including organ meats), egg yolk, poultry, and seafood (tuna, shrimp, clams, oysters), and brewer's yeast.
- ✿ Eat foods high in vitamin C, which enhance iron absorption.
- ✿ Avoid foods and medicines that inhibit iron absorption—coffee, carbonated sodas, black tea, dairy, and antacids.
- ✿ Calcium blocks iron absorption. Avoid eating calcium-rich foods when eating iron- rich foods.
- ✿ Drink Nettle tea.
- ✿ Yellow dock tincture helps iron absorption.
- ✿ Floradix® natural liquid iron supplement with whole food concentrates.
- ✿ Cook in a cast-iron pot.

Homeopathic Medicines

- ✿ *Ferrum metallicum* is indicated for anemia associated with exhaustion, weakness, pale skin, and feeling worse after physical activity. It can also be used when there is swelling of lower legs.
- ✿ *Calcarea phosphorica* is considered a good general remedy for anemia in pregnancy. It is useful for weakness and cold hands and feet. As part of every tissue in the body, it is vital for healthy bones, blood, tissue, and growth.
- ✿ Take *Ferrum metallicum* 6X alternating with *Calcarea phosphorica* 6X, 3 pellets every other day. Can be taken daily for more severe anemia.

ANXIETY

See also *Grief and Sorrow*

During pregnancy it is common for women to experience worry about many things including having a healthy baby, going through childbirth, and becoming a parent. For some mothers-to-be, it can be extremely anxiety provoking, and a woman can become overwhelmed which can interfere with daily activities. At Stanford's Center for Neuroscience in Women's Health, studies found that anxiety can affect up to 20 percent of pregnant women. Women with clinical anxiety are more at risk for premature delivery and postpartum depression. Anxious feelings stem from pre-existing complaints of the past, as well as current situations, including unexpected results from a test, history of abuse, and past birth traumas. (See "Fear and Anxiety: The Nocebo Effect" in "Introduction to Natural Pregnancy" and "Birth Trauma and PTSD" in Chapter 4.)

Care and Treatment

When complaints begin to interrupt sleep or daily activities, consider additional measures for relief. Ask for help from others including family, your healthcare practitioner, and mental health professionals. More severe cases of anxiety are treated with psychotherapy, and even medications. However, many women are resistant to taking medications, especially during pregnancy, and prefer to begin with a more natural approach.

Homeopathic Medicines

Homeopathic remedies work well for alleviating acute anxiety. Consider a consultation with a professional homeopath for relief of chronic suffering and emotional distress.

- ❁ *Aconitum napellus* is useful for relieving feelings of anxiety and panic stemming from a sudden event such as an accident, a fright, or a shocking event. Indications for *Aconite* are nervousness, agitation, and fast heartbeat. In Los Angeles during the 1994 earthquake, it is said that all the local homeopathic pharmacies sold out of *Aconite.*

- ❁ *Arsenicum album* is indicated for anxiety accompanied by restlessness and the desire for company. Worries can vary, from the fear of getting into a car accident to a fixation with locking the doors in the home at night to prevent intruders, and may include a tendency toward obsessive compulsive reactions. She can feel chilly and worse at midnight.

❀ *Ignatia amara* is the main remedy for loss and grief. She may be hysterical with complaints of nervous headache, a sensation of a lump in the throat, numbness, intermittent sighing, and uncontrollable weeping.

❀ *Gelsemium* is recommended for fear that manifests as trembling, fright, and anticipatory anxiety. Along with the anxiety there may be weakness, diarrhea, and dizziness. *Gelsemium* is also well known as a remedy for flu symptoms.

❀ *Rescue Remedy*, made from Bach Flower Essences, is excellent for stressful and anxious times. Bach Flower remedies were developed by Dr. Edward Bach, and can be used to treat emotional imbalances. Place 2 drops in a glass of water, sip as needed.

BLADDER INFECTIONS

Bladder infections, also known as cystitis or urinary tract infection (UTI) is a bacterial infection of any part of the urinary system, including the urethra, bladder, ureters, and kidneys. Because of the female anatomy, women are more at risk. The uterus is situated on top of the bladder. As the baby grows during pregnancy, the enlarged uterus can interfere with the urine flow from the bladder. UTIs may also be due to hormonal changes in the body, as well as the demands on the kidney to filter the blood, which may be increased in volume by 50 percent. Symptoms include pain, burning, cramping, and discomfort when urinating, as well as urgency. The urine may have a strong odor. It can appear bloody or cloudy. Some women have no symptoms at all. It is best to notify your practitioner if you have ongoing symptoms, and especially if they are accompanied by fever, chills, and back pain.

Care and Treatment
Conventional Treatment
UTIs are checked through urinalysis and culture. Practitioners usually prescribe a 3 to 7 day course of antibiotics.

Prevention

✿ Fully empty your bladder. After urinating, while sitting on the toilet, take your hand and lift your belly off your bladder, as you may be able to urinate a little more.

✿ Urinate when you have the urge. Wipe from the front to the back.

✿ Increase fluids, so that you are urinating many times throughout the day.

✿ Eat healthy. Avoid coffee, tea, sugar, refined foods, and alcohol.

✿ Urinate before and after intercourse. Avoid intercourse if you have UTI symptoms.

✿ Use clean cotton underwear and avoid synthetic fabrics and tight pants.

✿ Avoid irritating products, especially commercial soaps, douches, and feminine hygiene products.

✿ Avoid prolonged baths.

✿ Remember to do your exercise, including Kegel exercises. This strengthens the pelvic floor muscles which support the bladder (at least 40 per day, in groups of 10).

Home Treatment

✿ Keep your trunk warm. Use a hot water bottle on the belly.

✿ Get adequate rest and exercise.

✿ Drink unsweetened cranberry juice.

✿ Take apple cider vinegar: 1 tablespoon in water, twice per day.

✿ Increase Vitamin C: 1,000 mg or more per day if having symptoms.

✿ If symptoms persist or worsen, see your practitioner.

Homeopathic Medicines

✿ *Cantharis* is one of most common remedies to use for acute bladder infections as well as kidney infections. The indications for *Cantharis* are severe burning before, during, and after urination. Each drop of urine passes as if it were scalding water. There is a constant desire to urinate. There can be large amounts of blood in the urine, and mood is anxious and agitated.

✿ *Pulsatilla* should be considered as a first line homeopathic medicine for general bladder irritation during pregnancy. There can be urinary frequency and incontinence. The mood is weepy, and there is a desire for fresh air.

✿ *Sepia* is known for its treatment for a heaviness, or bearing-down sensation in the pelvic region associated with prolapse of the bladder (cystocele). This can lead to urinary incontinence. She can be easily irritated, and feels better with exercise.

✿ *Staphysagria* helps in bladder infections accompanied by the frequent urge to urinate and a sensation of urine dripping in the urethra. Burning sensations in the urethra may persist. *Staphysagria* is indicated for bladder infections after sex and earned its reputation for treatment of "honeymoon cystitis." It is also for bladder infections following sexual abuse. Emotionally, there is a tendency toward suppressing emotions, especially anger.

BREECH AND TURNING BABIES

During labor, the optimal position for baby is head down. At some point during pregnancy, most babies are in a breech position, which means baby's feet or bottom are in the pelvis. Ultimately, most turn toward the end of pregnancy. Breech position accounts for 4 percent of all pregnancies at term. Since doctors are no longer trained in breech deliveries, most breech babies will be delivered by cesarean section. In the past, most were delivered vaginally.

There are things to do that may help the baby turn into a more optimal position. Of the three presentations, Frank Breech is considered the most favorable, when baby's bottom presents first with his feet by the head. Footling Breech is when one or both feet present first, and Complete Breech is when baby is sitting cross legged, with his feet near the buttocks.

Care and Treatment
Prevention

✿ The pelvic tilt exercise benefits everyone, especially in pregnancy. It encourages baby to stay in an optimal position or to move into one for labor, which is when baby is facing mom's back with his back against mom's belly. Perform 40 every day in sets of 10. (See "Exercise" in Chapter 1 and spinningbabies.com.)

❀ Chiropractic preventive care is recommended during pregnancy, as it is known for easing delivery. The Webster technique relaxes the pelvic structures and ligaments in pregnant women with a success rate of 82 percent in turning babies from breech position.

Conventional Treatment

The standard medical approach utilizes an external cephalic version (a procedure used to turn a fetus from a breech position) performed by an obstetrician who places his or her hands on mother's belly to turn the baby. This is performed in a hospital and requires fetal monitoring, ultrasound, and medications. Most women prefer to try the natural approaches before resorting to the external version.

Home and Natural Treatments

❀ Slant board exercise: Place a sturdy board with one end on the floor and the other on a sofa. Carefully lie on the board with your head lower than your feet. Do this for 10 to 15 minutes, three times per day. It is best to do this on an empty stomach.

❀ Place a bag of frozen peas at the top of the belly (by baby's head). This can be done on a slant board, or in a warm bath with the upper belly out of the water. Babies move away from cold (who wouldn't?) toward warmth.

❀ Swimming: Do a headstand in the water with somersaults.

❀ Music: Place headphones with soothing music on the lower belly. Babies gravitate to sound.

❀ Acupuncture can be successful, as can acupressure and the use of moxibustion, a technique in which the herb, mugwort, is made into a small cone shape and placed over an acupuncture point and lit to burn for a few seconds. The heat generated stimulates the energy flow which is meant to address complaints and improve general health.

❀ Homeopathy: *Pulsatilla* is known for turning babies. The woman may be weepy and depressed. *Pulsatilla* 30C, 3 pellets three times per day for 3 days.

CESAREAN SECTION

See "Postpartum Wound Care" on page 169

CHORIONIC VILLUS SAMPLING (CVS)

See *Wound Care*

CONSTIPATION AND DIGESTIVE ISSUES

See also *Heartburn; Hemorrhoids*

Due to hormonal changes in the body during pregnancy, food is digested more slowly and can lead to constipation, a common complaint in pregnant women. This can also be a problem in later months with pressure from the growing uterus. Straining can cause hemorrhoids, another common problem.

Care and Treatment

Conventional Treatment

In addition to the measures below, practitioners may prescribe fiber supplements and stool softeners. Consider diet and lifestyle changes before resorting to medications.

Prevention and Home Treatment

- ❀ Eat healthy, and include plenty of fresh fruits and vegetables in your diet. (See "Nutrition and Pregnancy" in Chapter 1.)
- ❀ Include organic prunes (stewed or juice).
- ❀ Drink 6-8 glasses of water per day.
- ❀ Drink warm fluids, including homemade broth, blackstrap molasses (1 tablespoon in warm water), tea, fresh lemonade with honey to taste.
- ❀ Keep moving—exercise on a regular basis.
- ❀ Use the toilet when you feel the urge, rather than postpone it.
- ❀ When on the toilet, place your feet up on a stool (or trash bin) to simulate a comfortable squatting position.
- ❀ Avoid iron supplements, which are constipating (they may be in your prenatal vitamin). Instead, consider more herbal choices (see "Anemia").

Homeopathic Medicines

❀ *Arsenicum album* is worth mentioning in this list because some women experience diarrhea during pregnancy. Known as the classic food poisoning remedy, *Arsenicum* is indicated for loose stool following eating, with offensive diarrhea including undigested food. She can feel exhausted. She prefers company and feels chilly, but improves with warmth.

❀ *Nux vomica* is useful for constipation when there is much straining, with passing small quantity of stool, but feeling incomplete. The stool can be difficult and painful. *Nux vomica* is indicated for women who lead sedentary lives, work too much, and are accustomed to a lifestyle of drinking coffee, wine, and rich and high-seasoned foods.

❀ *Pulsatilla* can be used for changeable bowels, such as diarrhea alternating with constipation. There can be burning, smarting, and rawness in the anus after stool. She is sensitive to rich foods. Her mood is weepy and she likes to be consoled.

❀ *Sepia* is for constipation where the stool is difficult to pass with straining. The stool may be covered with mucus, and she may feel a ball, or bearing-down sensation, in the anus. Her mood appears indifferent to loved ones and she is easily offended. She can be sad and weepy, with an aversion to company.

CYSTITIS

See *Bladder Infections*

DEPRESSION

See *Anxiety, Grief and Sorrow*

DIARRHEA

See *Constipation and Digestive Issues*

EDEMA

During pregnancy it is common for women to experience swelling, also known as edema. This is due to the body producing, and then retaining, more fluids. In addition, as the uterus grows it puts pressure on the pelvic veins, causing blood to pool below the knees. Late in pregnancy, the lower legs, face, and hands can be more swollen, and some women are also susceptible, especially in warmer weather. Mild swelling in pregnancy is common, but reasons to contact your healthcare provider include swelling in one leg (which may be a sign of a blood clot) or severe or sudden onset of swelling. The latter could be a sign of a serious condition known as preeclampsia, which is characterized by high blood pressure in pregnancy associated with protein in the urine, headaches, and blurred vision.

Care and Treatment

Home Treatment

* Drink plenty of water throughout the day.
* Eat healthy; including a high protein diet as suggested by the Brewer Pregnancy Diet (see Chapter 1).
* Avoid prolonged standing or sitting and change position at least hourly.
* Avoid crossing the legs when seated.
* When sitting, elevate legs if swollen.
* Exercise regularly.
* Go swimming. The water pressure helps disperse the additional fluid.
* Avoid tight socks.
* Sleep on your left side to allow improved blood flow.
* *Sulphur* is a well-known skin remedy and is useful for swelling of the lower extremities during pregnancy. According to Dr. Richard Moskowitz, "*Sulphur* is an important remedy in late pregnancy, when the dramatically increased blood volume tends to be associated with excessive heat production and other symptoms referable to it, notably edema, hypertension, insomnia, and the like."

EMOTIONAL UPSET

See *Anxiety; Grief and Sorrow*

EPIDURAL

See "Postpartum Wound Care" on page 169

EPISIOTOMY

See "Postpartum Wound Care" on page 169

GENITAL HERPES

Genital herpes is a common infection, and it is estimated that up to 25 percent of pregnant women have experienced outbreaks. Referred to as herpes simplex virus 2, it is distinguished from herpes simplex virus 1, which is a common cause of cold sores or fever blisters on the lip. The concern is the transmission of the virus from the mother to her newborn, although even then it is rare. When neonatal herpes does occur, it is a serious illness and can lead to such conditions as encephalitis and meningitis, with a 60 percent mortality rate.

It is considered more of a threat to babies in women who have their first outbreak late in pregnancy. The latter is usually uncommon in women with monogamous partners. Rates are lowest in women who have experienced outbreaks before pregnancy, or during early pregnancy. This is because mother's body has had time to develop antibodies which help protect the baby, which can take twelve weeks. After the initial herpes infection, symptoms tend to be milder. However, general complaints can include fever, painful genital ulcer, itching, swollen lymph glands in the groin, inguinal lymph glands, and headaches.

Women with recurrent outbreaks should consider constitutional treatment with a holistic practitioner, possibly a homeopath, to help treat the complaints and strengthen her immune system to decrease the severity and frequency of outbreaks. Below are some homeopathic suggestions that are valuable for acute infection.

Care and Treatment

Conventional Treatment

The medical approach includes use of antiviral therapy to all women who experience their first outbreak of genital herpes in pregnancy, regardless of early or late pregnancy. Treatment is also indicated for women who have active recurrent infections. Suppressive antiviral therapy begins at 36 weeks and is continued until delivery. Cesarean section is recommended for women with active genital lesions or early signs of an impending outbreak. Cesarean is not recommended for women with a history of herpes, who do not have an outbreak during labor.

Home Treatment

Many women with a history of recurrent outbreaks prefer to take preventive natural measures when possible. Homeopathic medicines can be extremely helpful. It is recommended to consult with your healthcare practitioner, and consider the following suggestions:

- ❧ Reduce stress, including work and relationship-related stress. It is known that stressing the body can increase outbreaks.
- ❧ Get plenty of rest.
- ❧ Eat well. Avoid refined foods, coffee, sugar, chocolate, nuts, and grains.
- ❧ Boost the immune system with Vitamin C, garlic, and other immune support.
- ❧ Avoid sexual intercourse, tight underwear, and pants during an outbreak.

Homeopathic Medicines

- ❧ *Sepia* is a commonly used homeopathic medicine for many complaints for women including genital herpes. It is also indicated for cold sores (also a herpes virus) around the mouth. She can also complain of a feeling of heaviness in the pelvic organs, constipation, and fatigue. She feels better with exercise. She can be irritable and easily overwhelmed.
- ❧ *Natrum muriaticum* is also used for genital herpes outbreaks and fever blisters. She may also have complaints such as vaginal dryness and migraine headaches. Her disposition is sensitive and introverted with

a serious appearance. She may have suffered from prolonged grief and suppressed feelings. There is a craving for salty foods.

❧ *Phosphorus* is distinguished as a homeopathic medicine for herpes outbreaks in women who are generally fearful and anxious about health matters but are easily reassured. She is sympathetic to the needs of others. There is also a preference for cold drinks.

GRIEF AND SORROW (including Postpartum Depression)

See also *Anxiety*

Grief and sorrow can be likened to a wound of the heart and soul. Like any injury, it takes time to heal. Feelings of grief and sorrow can result from loss of a pregnancy or loss of a child, and can also include a period of postpartum depression following childbirth, when one mourns the loss of a former lifestyle. Following any difficult experience, it is normal to go through a period of pain and suffering.

Care and Treatment

Ask for help and support from friends, family, and professionals. Homeopathic medicines can help in dealing with difficult experiences in acute situations. A meeting with a professional for a constitutional remedy can alleviate symptoms in chronic cases.

Homeopathic Medicines

❧ *Ignatia amara* is the main remedy for loss, sorrow, and grief. It is indicated when sensations include a lump in the throat, sighing, and uncontrollable weeping. Nearly all my new mothers appreciate *Ignatia* sometime in the week or so following birth, and it can be used throughout the postpartum period.

❧ *Natrum muriaticum* is useful for the woman who suffers quietly and keeps her feelings to herself. She tends to be overly responsible and avoids company. She may have difficulty crying and may experience long periods of sadness following a loss. There can be a craving for salty foods, lemon, and ice cold drinks.

✿ *Phosphoric acidum*, also for grief, is indicated when a woman feels depleted and indifferent rather than sad. This is an excellent remedy for complaints of hair loss in the postpartum period especially when combined with the above indications. Symptoms improve following a short nap, and she may have a desire for refreshing fruit juices and carbonated drinks. She may also feel homesick and nostalgic.

✿ *Sepia* is used more often in the long-term stages following birth. The mom who could benefit from *Sepia* is feeling emotionally detached from her children and partner (and does not know why). She lacks energy and feels better when she exercises. She is conscientious about her responsibilities but worn out by caring for everyone; she feels like being alone and getting away from it all.

✿ *Bach Flower Essences* can be used in conjunction with homeopathic remedies. Bach Flower remedies were developed by Dr. Edward Bach, and can be used to treat emotional imbalances. Place 2 drops in a glass of water, sip as needed.

✿ *Star of Bethlehem* helps to relieve sadness associated with loss and grief. Also for post-traumatic stress.

✿ *Rescue Remedy* is a combination of five flower essences, including *Star of Bethlehem*. It can be used for sadness and grief associated with emergency situations and panic, such as that following an accident or when receiving unexpected test results.

HEARTBURN

As pregnancy progresses, many women experience heartburn especially in the second and third trimester. Often referred to as indigestion or acid reflux, it is caused by the hormonal changes which affect the digestive tract as well as the growing baby that crowds the abdomen, pushing up in the stomach. This condition is characterized by a myriad of symptoms such as burning, irritation, regurgitation, discomfort, burping, distention, nausea, and fullness—all of which can be felt in the stomach and extend upward through the chest and throat. Indigestion can also interfere with sleep.

Care and Treatment
Conventional Treatment

In addition to general preventive measures, practitioners commonly prescribe antacids. However, many women prefer to try home remedies and natural medical choices first to avoid any unwarranted side effects. Consult with your practitioner if symptoms persist, and before taking antacids.

Prevention and Home Treatment

❁ Eat slowly and in small amounts throughout the day, rather than consuming three large meals.

❁ Eat healthy and avoid greasy, spicy, and fatty foods.

❁ Take plain yogurt after a meal to help soothe the gut.

❁ Drink fluids in between meals, not with food.

❁ Avoid lying down immediately after eating.

❁ Sleep elevated on several pillows, if needed.

❁ Avoid tight-fitting clothes.

❁ A hot water bottle placed on the belly can be soothing.

❁ Eat raw almonds (just a few) which can soothe and neutralize stomach acid.

❁ Drink coconut water or ginger tea.

❁ Try apple cider vinegar: 1 tablespoon mixed in water.

❁ Drink herbal pregnancy teas for heartburn with Red Raspberry Leaf, Spearmint/Peppermint, Ginger root, Slippery Elm Bark, and Chamomile.

Homeopathic Medicines

❁ *Carbo vegetabilis* is good for complaints of fullness, bloating, and burning especially after eating rich foods. Digestion is slow and she feels better with burping and passing gas. There is a desire for open air or a fan.

❁ *Lycopodium* is a wonderful digestive remedy for such complaints as sour upset stomach, distension, and gas. There can be belching with burning in the throat lasting for hours. She feels hungry at night, but even slight eating leads to fullness. Loud rumbling in the tummy with a craving for sweets. She is worse from 4 to 8 P.M., with complaints worse on the right side.

❀ *Nux vomica* is indicated for women who have heartburn because they tend to overindulge in food and drinks, including coffee and rich and spicy foods. They suffer from nausea, vomiting, sour burps, and a heavy knot in the stomach. Known to occur in type A personalities, women who respond well to *Nux vomica* can be constipated and feel better after a bowel movement and a good night's sleep.

❀ *Pulsatilla* can be used for heartburn after a meal where there is great tightness, and she must loosen clothing. She is obliged to eat a small amount at a time, with sensitivity to fatty and rich foods, and is rarely thirsty. She feels warm and enjoys the fresh air. She is weepy and needs reassurance.

❀ *Robinia* is for severe burning and acidity along the whole GI tract. There is sour acid reflux and burping. She has difficulty sleeping because the acidity is worse at night while lying down.

❀ *Sepia* is prescribed for heartburn where there is a sinking feeling in the stomach, with burning and acidity. There can also be nausea with the smell of food. She craves vinegar and pickles and feels better with vigorous exercise. She is worse in the late afternoon and can be easily irritated.

HEMORRHOIDS (PILES)

See also *Constipation and Digestive Issues; Varicose Veins*

Hemorrhoids are varicose veins in the rectal area caused by pressure from the growing baby in the uterus. They can be aggravated during delivery, and also with straining due to constipation, which is another common complaint during pregnancy. Hemorrhoids are either internal or external—the latter look (and feel) like a pile of grapes in the anal area. They can be painful with swelling, itching, burning, bleeding, and generalized discomfort. However, sometimes there is no pain at all. They usually subside following delivery.

Care and Treatment
Conventional Treatment
In addition to the home treatment suggestions below, the standard medical approach is to prescribe fiber supplements, stool softener, and over-the-counter hemorrhoid creams as needed.

Home Treatment
❀ Keep the bowels moving—eat plenty of fruits and vegetables and stay hydrated.

❀ Stay physically active on a daily basis.

❀ Kegel exercises and Pelvic Tilts improve circulation. Perform both 40 per day in sets of 10.

❀ Avoid prolonged sitting or standing.

❀ Place your feet on a stool (or trash can) by the toilet for bowel movements. Avoid straining.

❀ Keep the anal area clean. Gently wipe after each bowel movement with moistened toilet paper. Pat dry.

❀ Relieve discomfort with a warm bath, ice packs, and sitting on a doughnut-shaped pillow.

Homeopathic Medicines
❀ *Aesculus hippocastanum* is a common remedy for engorged burning hemorrhoids with backache. The rectum feels full of small sticks. *Aesculus* is also found in topical homeopathic hemorrhoid creams combined with *Hamamelis*.

Hamamelis virginica (Witch-hazel) is a well-known hemorrhoid medicine used in both standard and holistic medicine. It is known as *Arnica* for the rectum. It can be used topically or orally. Soak cotton pads (or sanitary napkin) in witch hazel astringent and apply directly to anal area or apply a topical homeopathic cream (or ointment). It can also be found combined with *Aesculus*. Also available in suppositories. When taken orally it is indicated for a sore, raw anus with hemorrhoids that bleed profusely.

✿ *Nux vomica* is used for hemorrhoids with additional symptoms of constipation with straining at stool but passage in small quantity. The hemorrhoids itch and are very painful. Her mood can be angry and impatient. Well known for treating the effects of doing "too much," such as eating too much food or working too much, it is also indicated for the typical Type A personality, full of ambition and stress. *Nux vomica* is also useful for varicose veins.

✿ *Pulsatilla* is indicated for bleeding hemorrhoids with itching, smarting, and rawness. Varicose veins are swollen, red, and painful. The veins can appear blue from the knees to the ankles. Her symptoms can be changeable, including symptoms from constipation to diarrhea. She is intolerant of warm stuffy rooms, desires fresh air, and is prone to be emotional and weepy.

✿ *Sepia* is a well-known remedy for hemorrhoids and varicose veins in pregnancy. The hemorrhoids prolapse (slip down) and are worse with walking. She may also feel a ball sensation in the rectum. Pains shoot up in the rectum and vagina. *Sepia* is also indicated for distended, engorged varicose veins of both the leg and vulvar (labial) region. She is irritable and complains of feeling drained, and feels better with vigorous exercise.

✿ *Sulphur* is used for hemorrhoids which are hot, burning, and aggravated by a warm bath. The varicose veins of the leg are distended and engorged, and are worse when standing. *Sulphur* is also indicated for distended pelvic blood vessels (vulvar area). She is heat intolerant, may have redness around the anus, and passes foul smelling gas.

HERPES

See *Genital Herpes*

INDIGESTION

See *Heartburn*

INFERTILITY

See "A Note on Chronic and Severe Illnesses" on page 123

Many women who have difficulty conceiving or staying pregnant respond well to holistic treatments including homeopathy. Since there are many homeopathic medicines and each person is treated as an individual, fertility treatment with homeopathy is beyond the scope of this book. Following a comprehensive and detailed consultation, a homeopathic medicine is chosen that is specific for the patient and is meant to stimulate the body to heal itself, strengthen her constitution, and address any ongoing conditions. In my medical practice, I have witnessed dozens of women conceive and have a normal pregnancy after receiving a constitutional medicine.

IRON DEFICIENCY ANEMIA

See *Anemia*

ITCHING
(Pruritic Urticarial Papules and Plaques of Pregnancy [PUPPP])

During the third trimester, some pregnant mothers experience Pruritic Urticarial Papules and Plaques of Pregnancy (PUPPP), an extremely itchy and bumpy rash that begins on the belly around the umbilical region within the stretch marks and spreads on the trunk and downward to the thighs. It disappears after birth. Not considered dangerous but annoying, PUPPP is more common in first-time mothers, women with excessive weight gain, and those carrying multiples. Although the cause is not known, it may be linked to insufficient detoxification in the liver. Cholestasis, a condition which interferes with the flow of bile in the liver, is another complaint in pregnancy that also presents with itching. What distinguishes this from PUPPP is that the itching with cholestasis is intense, especially on the palms of the hands and soles of the feet. In addition it can also be accompanied by common liver symptoms such as jaundice, dark urine, and light stools. PUPPP is considered a benign self-limiting condition, whereas cholestasis is problematic and can lead to prematurity or fetal distress.

Care and Treatment
Conventional Treatment
Practitioners usually prescribe topical steroid creams and oral antihistamines. Many pregnant women are concerned about possible side effects and prefer to begin with more natural applications, some of which are listed below.

Home Treatment
- An oatmeal bath can be soothing.
- Use cold compresses.
- Grandpa's Pine Tar Soap has helped many pregnant women. Use while showering.
- *Dandelion Root* (*Taraxacum officinale*) is a well-known herb for the liver that has been used for medicinal purposes including with pregnant women for generations. It contains many vitamins (A, B, C, and D) and minerals (iron, potassium, and zinc). Added to salads or made as a tea, dandelion, is used for skin conditions, as a liver cleanser, and for upset stomach, heartburn, and edema. Herbalists recommend consuming a small amount of dandelion root throughout pregnancy as it may minimize or prevent constipation, gestational diabetes, or preeclampsia (toxemia).
- Eat healthy and avoid refined foods and sugar.
- Consult with a homeopath or other holistic practitioner who can offer individualized treatment after taking a detailed history and physical.

MASTITIS

Mastitis is an infection or inflammation of the breast. Mastitis can be extremely painful and is usually associated with hard, swollen, engorged breasts. There can also be a discharge from the nipple. In my practice, after trying the home treatments and homeopathic medicines below, we rarely need to resort to antibiotics. If you experience severe pain with breastfeeding, fever (higher than 100.6°F), flu-like symptoms (chills, body ache), or red streaks in the breast, consult your practitioner immediately.

Care and Treatment

Prevention and Home Treatment

To prevent engorgement, usually a common cause of mastitis:

- ✿ Nurse frequently, at least every 1 to 2 hours during the day and up to 3-hour stretches at night. Begin by nursing at least 15 minutes or longer on each side.
- ✿ Use breast pumps if your newborn is not feeding as often as two hours.
- ✿ Cold compresses between feedings may reduce swelling and congestion, and improve milk flow. Wrap in cloth, and place on the breast and underarms, avoiding the nipple or areola. Use for 15 to 20 minutes every 1 to 2 hours if needed for swelling.
- ✿ Warm compresses can be used just prior to breastfeeding or pumping to help your milk let down if you are engorged. Moist heat, such as a warm, wet cloth, is preferable. Avoid using warm compresses for more than five minutes as they can increase swelling.
- ✿ Gently massage breasts while taking a warm shower or bath, immersing breasts in a basin of warm water, or using a hot water bottle wrapped in a wet cloth.
- ✿ Place a few drops of olive oil on the breasts (avoid the nipple) while doing gentle breast massage prior to breast feeding.
- ✿ Use cabbage leaves for mastitis. Personally I used raw green cabbage leaves to help relieve fullness and sore nipples in between feedings. Trust me, it feels soothing! Clean the inner leaves of a green cabbage and place on breasts inside bra. They can be room temperature or chilled. Change every two hours or when wilted.
- ✿ Get plenty of rest and stay around the house, including taking naps with baby.
- ✿ Nursing bras or sports bras without underwires may be helpful for support.
- ✿ Avoid binding the breasts, which can lead to plugged ducts.
- ✿ Eat healthy and increase fluids.

❀ Use colloidal silver, a broad spectrum bactericide that can be used to maintain a strong immune system or can be used as a first line of defense. In my practice, we use colloidal silver whenever we suspect an infection, including mastitis.

❀ Check baby for tongue-tie which can cause painful breasts (see "Newborn Conditions")

Conventional Treatment

The standard prescribed care for pain and swelling is an anti-inflammatory drug, such as ibuprofen, or a stronger pain medication. In the case of a moderate to severe infection, antibiotics are prescribed. Nystatin may be given if your doctor suspects a yeast infection (thrush) on the nipple.

Homeopathic Medicines

❀ *Belladonna* is indicated when breasts are red, hot, swollen, and very tender. Symptoms can come on suddenly, and may be accompanied by high fever. Often pain occurs on the right side, with a throbbing sensation. The breast is extremely sensitive to touch or being jarred, with streaks radiating from the nipple.

❀ *Bryonia* is helpful in relieving breasts that are hot, painful, hard, and engorged. Symptoms may include stitching pains that are greatly aggravated by any motion, as well as a dry feeling and irritable mood.

❀ *Calendula officinalis* ointment or cream. Use prior to childbirth for several weeks, and in the first weeks of nursing. *Calendula* is an excellent natural topical and will help condition nipples and minimize cracking. Wash off before nursing.

❀ *Castor equi* is recommended for nipples with painful cracks or ulcers, and for extremely tender, swollen breasts that are sensitive to clothing and that feel worse when going down stairs. Breasts may also itch with redness of the areola.

❀ *Hepar sulphuris calcareum (Hepar sulph)* is a useful remedy for boils and abscesses in general, as well as for sore and cracked nipples, especially for pus-forming organisms. The woman's mood is irritable, and she tends to be chilly.

✿ *Phytolacca* is indicated for inflamed or swollen breasts that are also full of lumps. Nipples may be cracked and excoriated, and the mother will often experience intense suffering on putting child to breast, with pain radiating from the nipple all over the body. She may also have a sore throat with swollen glands.

✿ *Pulsatilla* is a versatile remedy used to prevent breast engorgement. *Pulsatilla* also helps to dry up mother's milk when weaning. Recommended for women whose mood is changeable and weepy.

✿ *Silica.* I use this remedy routinely after birth for several days to prevent or minimize sore nipples. It is recommended to relieve soreness and cracks on the nipples, accompanied by sharp, splinter-type pain (extending from breast to shoulder), and/or inflamed breast with constant burning.

MILK SUPPLY

Reasons for low milk supply include stress, fatigue, poor nutrition, inadequate water intake, infrequent nursing, nipple confusion from bottle or pacifier, supplementation with formula, or anatomical conditions with mother's breast or tongue-tie in newborns (see "Newborn Conditions"). Many mothers jump to conclusions about their milk supply; however, if your baby is gaining weight while exclusively on breast milk, then your milk supply is probably adequate.

Care and Treatment
Conventional Treatment

Prescription medications like Reglan can be used to increase milk supply. Most of my patients prefer to use the plethora of home remedies and natural treatments available rather than beginning with prescription medication.

Homeopathic Medicines

✿ *Lac defloratum* helps restore flow of milk when there is deficient production. Often the low milk supply is due to small atrophic breasts. The patient who responds well to *Lac defloratum* tends to become strongly fatigued and worn out, is often allergic to milk, and has a history of migraines.

✿ *Pulsatilla* can increase milk production when it is deficient, and restore milk supply after a breast infection.

✿ *Ricinus communis* is used to increase the quantity of milk in nursing women. It is indicated in women with large breasts. There may also be diarrhea.

Herbal Remedies

In addition to homeopathic medicines, herbs can increase milk supply. These are known as galactagogues and have been used for centuries in many cultures. Unlike homeopathics, herbal remedies may carry side effects. For this reason, I recommend you start with herbal tea. See your practitioner or lactation consultant if you are not getting the desired results.

✿ *Mother's Milk Tea®*, which contains fenugreek and other herbs, helps boost milk supply. As a tea, it is a milder galactagogue, but can still work effectively. Drink several cups per day as needed, either warm or cooled. Fenugreek is commonly used to increase milk supply and has been known to work very quickly. Employed for centuries in Ayurvedic and Chinese medicine, fenugreek's many indications include improving metabolism, managing diabetes, and reducing cholesterol. If you have a tendency to hypoglycemia or a history of diabetes, monitor blood sugar levels closely when taking fenugreek, as it can affect blood sugar levels.

✿ *Rescue Remedy* (Bach Flower Essence) can be helpful in triggering the letdown reflex and is also known for its calming influence during stressful times. If feeling overwhelmed, *Rescue Remedy* can help with relaxation, which will increase milk flow. Place 4 drops in a drink prior to pumping or nursing.

MISCARRIAGE

See "Miscarriage" in "Homeopathic Medicines for Labor" on page 168

MORNING SICKNESS

See *Nausea and Vomiting*

NAUSEA AND VOMITING

A common complaint during pregnancy is nausea, sometimes with vomiting, also known as *morning sickness*. It affects up to half of women usually during the first trimester, and does not occur only in the morning. Believed to be due to hormonal changes, it has also been linked to a mother's emotional state. It can also be accompanied by increased sensitivity to odors, especially of food. Morning sickness increases in women who have a history of motion sickness, migraines, poor nutrition, and nausea with previous pregnancies.

Care and Treatment

Call your healthcare provider for continued or severe nausea, vomiting, fainting, and inability to eat or drink for 24 hours. Signs of early dehydration include dark urine, infrequent urination, and dry mouth.

Home Treatment

- ❀ Ask someone else to cook if sensitive to odors.
- ❀ Eat crackers upon waking.
- ❀ Take prenatal vitamins with food.
- ❀ Avoid triggers such as strong odors, rich foods, and overeating. Heated foods have more odors.
- ❀ Drink fluids and eat frequently, but in small quantities.
- ❀ Add ginger to warm drinks. Grate ginger into hot water for tea. This can interact with anti-coagulants, so ask your healthcare provider before using. Indicated when feeling chills.
- ❀ Peppermint in cold drinks can help digestion, but avoid mint if taking homeopathic medicine as it can antidote.
- ❀ Drink Red Raspberry Leaf tea (only during second half of pregnancy).
- ❀ Provide fresh air.
- ❀ Vitamin B6, 25 mg, three times per day with water.
- ❀ Acupressure points are helpful, including wrist bands.

Homeopathic Medicines

❀ *Colchicum* can be used for morning sickness that is worse from the thought of food as well as the smell of cooked food, including fish, meat, and eggs. She has a keen sense of smell to any odor. She is worse from motion.

❀ *Ipecacuanha* is soothing for constant nausea with increased salivation. She is worse from motion, lying down, and does not feel any better after vomiting. There can be an aversion to food including the smell. Can be alternated with *Sepia*.

❀ *Nux vomica* is for nausea associated with burping and retching following eating. Nausea is especially worse in the morning and after eating. There may be a tendency to overeat, but a relief with vomiting. She is over-sensitive to light, sound, odors, and the cold. She can be dizzy with the nausea, constipated, and may feel angry and impatient.

❀ *Pulsatilla* is for nausea with heartburn. She is sensitive to eating fatty foods, and is averse to drinking. She feels better outside, prefers cool air, and is worse in the heat. Her mood can be weepy and she desires conso-lation and reassurance.

❀ *Sepia* is for constant nausea, which is worse in the morning and late afternoon. The nausea is intensified by the thought or smell of food. There is a craving for vinegar, sours, and pickles. If she is able, she feels better with strong exercise. She may feel indifferent about the pregnancy, easily irritated, and tired.

❀ *Symphoricarpus racemosa* is for severe and continuous nausea and vom-iting (hyperemesis gravidarum). The thought and smell of food causes nausea, and the vomiting is intense. She is worse with motion, and feels relieved by lying quietly and still on her back. She has loss of appetite. Use this remedy when others fail.

❀ *Tabacum* is a well known remedy for motion sickness, with tremendous nausea that is worse from odors including food, exhaust, and chemicals. There can be violent vomiting accompanied with sweat. She feels better in fresh air, and after uncovering the belly and closing her eyes. Worse with motion.

NERVOUS PARTNERS AND GRANDPARENTS

In addition to mother's own feelings about pregnancy and having a baby, the concerns and worries that come from expectant fathers (and grandparents) can affect mother and her environment. Often these thoughts and feelings are apparent before labor, so homeopathic medicines can be used anytime. For many people who have no experience in labor and delivery, witnessing a birth can be anxiety provoking because it is a profound human experience. Especially during labor when sudden changes may occur, homeopathic medicines can be helpful in ensuring calm. With a well-chosen homeopathic medicine, one dose may be all that is needed.

Care and Treatment
Homeopathic Medicines

❧ *Aconitum napellus* is indicated following an event that happens suddenly. There are feelings of panic and fear, and racing heart rate. Common triggers can stem from an unexpected change in labor, difficult labor, or postpartum bleeding. Whether it is rational or not, typical thought patterns (which may or may not be verbalized) include, "She could die! Call an ambulance! Oh gosh!" Give one dose of *Aconitum* 30C or 200C.

❧ *Arsenicum album* is used for a partner who fears that he could lose his wife, on whom he is dependent. He appears concerned and restless, and paces back and forth. He is controlling and reports to the midwife or doctor minor details. His imagination can make a "mountain out of molehill," and he needs to be reassured that everything is going to be okay.

❧ *Gelsemium* is for the expectant father who greatly anticipates labor and delivery. He feels weak and he is shaky. During labor he may need to sit down because he may faint.

❧ *Phosphorus* is for the sympathetic partner who experiences the morning sickness and heartburn with his wife. Especially in labor, he has great fears and concerns about her suffering in labor. He too can easily panic.

❧ *Rescue Remedy* (Bach Flower Essence) is excellent for stressful and anxious times. If the homeopathic medicines are not available, *Rescue Remedy* can be used. Place 2 drops in a glass of water and sip.

NEWBORN CONDITIONS
(including Tongue-Tie)

Occasionally there are times when baby is born with conditions that require immediate attention. For newborn emergencies, your healthcare practitioner is trained to begin treatment. In addition, there are homeopathic medicines that can be used in conjunction with conventional methods, with great success. The more common conditions that may be seen following birth include difficulty breathing (asphyxia) and birth injuries. For more information on treatment options for newborn jaundice, umbilical cord care, blocked tear ducts, and more, see *Natural Baby and Childcare* (Hatherleigh Press, 2006).

It may take several hours for baby to establish a regular pattern of breathing following delivery. Commonly, nasal passages can be blocked from secretions which can be cleared with suctioning and a bulb syringe. Respiratory issues can lead to rapid breathing, chest congestion, and blue skin coloring—all of which require medical assessment.

Following a long and difficult birth, including need of forceps or cesarean section, baby may be injured during the process. General bruising and swelling of the head is not uncommon, including an occasional fractured collarbone (clavicle).

A relatively common condition known as tongue-tie (ankyloglossia or "anchored tongue") is found in newborns. Tongue-tie can impact breastfeeding and milk supply. In the past, newborns were checked for tongue-tie and treated when needed. Being tongue tied means the frenulum which is the thin cord or webbing that stretches from under the tongue to the floor of the mouth is too short or tight and limits the movement of the tongue. According to research, up to 15% of babies were found to have tongue tie. This condition, which occurs during development, is often found in other family members and is more common in boys than girls. In the past, all practitioners examined and treated newborns for tongue-tie because it could compromise breastfeeding, but also interferes with speech later on. It was known that midwives kept a sharp fingernail handy to sweep under the tongue to clip the extra tissue at birth.

When my first son was born he was tongue-tied which was diagnosed by my father, who was an ear, nose and throat surgeon. At the time I did not think much of it, as I was able to successfully breastfeed, and all seemed fine...so I thought.

However, as a teenager his dentist noted that in addition to having severe tongue-tie, his teeth were crowded and the roof of his mouth (palate) was narrowed. We subsequently learned about the consequences of tongue-tie.

Normally, the tongue should be able to easily move up to the roof of the mouth (palate). Being able to rest the tongue on the palate serves to shape and widen the mouth, jaw, and even facial features. This allows for more room for the teeth (including wisdom teeth). When the tongue is not able to move with ease, it leads to crowding of the teeth, speech problems, snoring, and even sleep apnea in adults. In order to try to breathe easier, the body compensates by jutting out the chin, leading to poor posture and neck and back pain. Conditions that lead to mouth breathing and sleep apnea can also be due to other conditions such as enlarged tonsils and adenoids. That was a lot of information in one dental visit! Within a short amount of time, my son underwent the procedure and was given specific exercises (myofunctional therapy) to keep the tongue mobile, avoid the tissue growing back, and improve breathing habits.

Following my experience, I now examine all newborns in our office for tongue-tie, and recommend that the frenulum be clipped when needed. At the newborn age, this is a simple procedure known as a frenotomy; no medication is needed. For older children and adults, the procedure, known as a frenulectomy (tongue-tie surgery), becomes more complex.

Care and Treatment
Homeopathic Medicines

- ✿ *Aconitum napellus*, known as SOS, is a well-known rescue medication following a sudden event. Consider *Aconite* for baby and family members following a traumatic birth with feelings of shock, fear, and anxiety.

- ✿ *Antimonium tartaricum* is indicated for lung and breathing conditions. These include chest congestion, great rattling of mucus in the chest with each breath, and wet cough (though unable to bring up much mucus). The infant may cry and have difficulty nursing. In addition, she may also have blue lips in severe cases and appear drowsy, weak, and pale. For any severe condition that impedes breathing, seek immediate medical attention.

✿ *Arnica Montana* is used for all bruises, swelling, and trauma to the newborn. Use after a frenotomy. In addition to baby, I use *Arnica* during the postpartum period for mothers.

PERINEAL TEAR

See "Postpartum Wound Care" on page 169

PILES

See *Hemorrhoids*

POSTPARTUM DEPRESSION

See *Grief and Sorrow*

PRURITIC URTICARIAL PAPULES AND PLAQUES OF PREGNANCY (PUPPP)

See *Itching*

RASH

See *Itching*

SURGERY (CESAREAN SECTION)

See "Postpartum Wound Care" on page 169

SWELLING

See *Edema*

TONGUE-TIE

See *Newborn Conditions*

VARICOSE VEINS

See also *Hemorrhoids*

Varicose veins are a common complaint due to the increased blood volume in pregnancy as well as pressure from the growing baby in the uterus, which cause the blood to accumulate in the veins. They are large, bulging, dark-red-to-purplish veins usually on the leg, and may be sore and painful, especially with prolonged standing or walking. Varicose veins in the vulvar region affect up to 10 percent of pregnant women and are thought to be hormonal. Varicose veins of the rectum are known as hemorrhoids. Varicose veins tend to be hereditary.

Care and Treatment

Prevention and Home Treatment

- ❧ Avoid straining, lifting, and carrying heavy objects.
- ❧ Loosen tight clothing.
- ❧ Compression stockings promote venous blood circulation. Discuss with your practitioner.
- ❧ Elevate legs when sitting and avoid crossing them.
- ❧ Be active and flex feet often.
- ❧ Take extra Vitamin C to strengthen veins.
- ❧ Keep weight in an optimal range.
- ❧ Apply witch-hazel cotton soaks to affected areas on the leg.
- ❧ For homeopathic treatment, see *Hemorrhoids*.

WOUND CARE
(Following Amniocentesis, Chorionic Villus Sampling (CVS), Epidural Anesthesia)

See also "Postpartum Wound Care" on page 169

Homeopathic medicines are extremely versatile and can aid healing following common procedures in pregnancy, as well as after birth itself. Amniocentesis, CVS, and Epidural Anesthesia use needle insertions, and require time for healing afterward.

Care and Treatment
Home Treatment

- ✿ Rest as indicated (and rest some more!)
- ✿ Use a hot water bottle on the belly when indicated.

Homeopathic Medicines

In general, following an amniocentesis, CVS or epidural, I prescribe both *Arnica* 30C and *Ledum* 30C. Use *Gelsemium* for nervousness before the procedure as needed. Take at least three times per day for 1-3 days. Upon improvement, taper and then discontinue.

- ✿ *Arnica montana* is the first medicine to use following invasive procedures and surgery. *Arnica* is an excellent treatment for trauma with complaints of bruising and soreness. Use *Arnica* after Chorionic villus sampling (CVS) and amniocentesis.
- ✿ *Gelsemium* can be used for anticipation and anxiety, before a procedure.
- ✿ *Hypericum perforatum* is excellent for injury to nerves, especially in the fingers, toes, nails, and spinal cord. The characteristic pains are shooting and sharp, and very sensitive to the touch. *Hypericum* is also indicated for puncture wounds following CVS, amniocentesis, and epidural spinal anesthesia.
- ✿ *Ledum palustre* is also recommended for puncture wounds with much swelling and inflammation, particularly when the inflamed area looks purple, puffy, and is cold to the touch. Similar to *Hypericum, Ledum* can be used following CVS, amniocentesis, and epidural spinal anesthesia.

Homeopathy for Childbirth

Labor Preparation

The last month of pregnancy is an ideal time to begin to wind down from professional duties and daily commitments (when possible). If you have not already started, it is important to take time out to prepare the "nest" for labor, as well as for welcoming baby. Now that you are almost at the home stretch, consider the following labor preparation techniques for increasing the chances of an easier delivery and postpartum period:

- Healthy nutrition is important throughout pregnancy and beyond (see Chapter 1)
- Keep moving! Continue practicing pelvic tilts.
- Practice exercises from childbirth class (if applicable).
- Take a breastfeeding class.
- Practice Kegel exercises.
- Consider perineal massage. Begin by week 37 (see Chapter 3).
- Drink Raspberry Leaf Tea, a well-known herb greatly esteemed during pregnancy. Brewed as a tea, it is commonly used in the second half of pregnancy. It is rich in vitamins and minerals, including vitamins C and E, and aids the assimilation of calcium and iron. Benefits include the following:
  - Tones the uterus
  - Eases morning sickness
  - Eases labor and reduces painful prolonged delivery
  - Optimizes contractions, making them more effective
  - May reduce risk of miscarriage and postpartum hemorrhage
- Pace yourself. Rest in between running errands.
- Have holistic medical visits with your healthcare provider. From a homeopath, chiropractor, acupuncturist to osteopath, receiving treatments for complaints and preventive medicine are known to ease birth and benefit both mother and baby (two for the price of one!).
- Enjoy this time for reflection.
- Go on a date with your spouse, and be intimate with him.

Homeopathic Pre-Labor Protocol for Easier Childbirth

Some practitioners recommend a pre-labor regimen to be used in the last trimester to ease childbirth. In a French double-blind study, homeopathic medicine has been shown to shorten labor time and help prevent or minimize the possibility of a difficult birth if taken daily, beginning at the ninth month. This protocol is indicated for women who feel anxious about the birth or anticipate their doctor would want to induce by a certain date. For women who have already experienced an easy or rapid labor, this protocol is not needed. Many of my patients have had great success using it and feel empowered by being able to participate in their healthcare. Personally I waited, as I wanted to see what my body would do on its own. Lo and behold, my first child was born at nearly 42 weeks. The following is adapted from the protocol:

- ❀ *Arnica* 12C or 30C (e.g. Monday)
- ❀ *Caulophyllum* 12C or 30C (e.g. Wednesday)
- ❀ *Cimicifuga* 12C or 30C (e.g. Friday)
- ❀ *Gelsemium* 12C or 30C (e.g. Saturday): Add *Gelsemium* for feelings of great anticipation and anxiety

Overdue: Natural Approach to Inducing Labor

Ina May Gaskin writes, "According to the midwifery model of care, women's bodies can generally be trusted to go into spontaneous labor." Although I am in favor of natural childbirth and letting Mother Nature take her course, I realize there are times when a woman may need assistance. Sometimes practitioners may suggest more natural ways to start labor. Be sure to discuss this with your practitioner before beginning. If your practitioner feels the need to induce, consider the following natural approaches.

Conventional Treatment

The medical model of care relies on the use of medications and methods used to induce labor, including sweeping the membranes, prostaglandins, and Pitocin. When a woman learns that there are natural approaches to inducing labor, many prefer to begin with them when possible (see Chapter 3).

Home Treatment

✿ Nipple stimulation in late pregnancy encourages the release of oxytocin, the same hormone that causes uterine contractions in labor. After baby is born, these contractions slow bleeding and help the uterus return to its normal pre-pregnancy size. Breast stimulation can be done manually or orally, through massaging both nipple and areola (in an effort to imitate a baby sucking). In the hospital setting, nipple stimulation is also done using an electric breastfeeding pump.

✿ Sexual intercourse is another way to induce labor, in that a man's semen provides a concentrated source of prostaglandins. This is the active ingredient in the medications Cervidil and Cytotec, which are used to induce labor by ripening the cervix. Unlike the synthetic prostaglandins, semen has no side effects (see Chapter 3, "Inducing Labor"). The effects of lovemaking are enhanced when combined with nipple stimulation.

✿ Walking: keep moving, but avoid overexertion.

✿ Castor oil is derived from the castor bean seed and has been used historically since the ancient Egyptians for such treatments as on skin and hair, and as a laxative. Known for its effects as a strong stimulant laxative, it has been used for generation to induce labor. Although the induction mechanisms are not known, the oil causes diarrhea by contracting the smooth muscles of the intestines which triggers uterine contractions, with the goal of inducing labor. The dosage used at The Farm Midwifery Center is 1 tablespoon of castor oil, which can be added to eggs or juice in the morning. If needed, repeat one hour later. It is important to stay hydrated, especially if there is diarrhea.

✿ Acupuncture and acupressure have been used for centuries. Many women have used the pressure points with great success to induce labor, much of which can be done at home. See a Chinese medicine practitioner. If this is not possible, there is also information online.

✿ Seek out chiropractic care, osteopathy, or cranial sacral therapy with a practitioner who is trained in pregnancy treatments.

✿ Evening primrose oil is used by some midwives to ripen the cervix.

❀ Eat pineapple, vinegar, and spicy foods. In Los Angeles, many women frequent a restaurant known for its special balsamic vinaigrette in their pregnancy salad to help jump-start labor contractions in overdue moms.
❀ Drink Red Raspberry Leaf Tea.

Homeopathic Medicines
Take each homeopathic medicine daily. Take 3 pellets under the tongue, separated by at least 30 minutes apart.
❀ *Arnica* 12C or 30C
❀ *Caulophyllum* 12C or 30C
❀ *Cimicifuga* 12C or 30C
❀ *Gelsemium* 12C or 30C
❀ *Pulsatilla* 12C or 30C

Homeopathic Medicines for Labor (Including Miscarriage)

I have seen wonderful results with homeopathic medicine for treating acute and chronic conditions. Homeopathy is safe, gentle, effective, and can be used in pregnancy, birth, and in the postpartum period. While many herbs and medications are contraindicated, homeopathy can also be used in the event of surgery, as in a cesarean section. While there are many medicines in our homeopathic *Materia Medica* for birth kits, the following are common choices that can be used by laypeople. In the "Guide to Homeopathic Medicines (Materia Medica)" on page 174, there is a full description of the labor remedies. Because there are many medicines for similar complaints, such as painful labor contractions, when deciding upon a homeopathic medicine, pay particular attention to the subtleties in the mental and emotional sphere as they can guide you in making the correct choice.

FALSE LABOR PAINS

During pregnancy, women experience Braxton-Hicks contractions, which are painless and occasional contractions of the belly. Closer to due date, they become more regular and frequent, enticing some women to believe that true labor has begun. Quite often false labor pains can be confused with true labor pains: the latter are stronger, more regular, and dilate the cervix in preparation for delivery.

Caulophyllum is the first choice remedy if unsure. Take up to three times per day if needed. If no response after 3 doses, discontinue.

- ❀ *Caulophyllum* is indicated for the last weeks of pregnancy for false labor pains. *Caulophyllum* is used only at the end of pregnancy. Her mood can be excitable, hysterical, and she may feel pain in the small joints of fingers and toes.
- ❀ *Cimicifuga* is for false labor pains that are spasmodic and painful. Her mood is dark and pessimistic.
- ❀ *Pulsatilla* is also for false labor pains, and her mood can also be excitable. However, she may be tearful, and need to be comforted and reassured. She is warm and feels better moving about slowly in the open air.

PREMATURE LABOR

Premature labor is when a woman goes into labor before 37 weeks of pregnancy. Contact your healthcare provider if you feel you are going into labor early.

Standard Treatment

In addition to bed rest, many women are placed on medications such as Magnesium sulfate which is given intravenously.

Homeopathic Medicines

The homeopathic medicines below can be used in conjunction with the standard approach. Begin with one dose of 30C and use up to three times per day.

- ❀ *Caulophyllum* is considered one of the most useful remedies for the prevention of premature labor due to weakness of the cervix. The pregnant woman feels weak yet with nervous excitement.
- ❀ *Cimicifuga* is indicated for premature labor without other indications.
- ❀ *Gelsemium* for premature contractions is indicated with feelings of weakness, trembling, and flu-like aches and pains.
- ❀ *Magnesia phosphorica* is a well-known medicine for menstrual cramps, but can also be used for labor pain, including premature labor. She may also have complaints of leg cramps, especially at night, due to a magnesium deficiency. She feels better with warmth (e.g. a hot water bottle) and pressure.

✿ *Pulsatilla* for premature labor can present with a weepy tearful mood. She prefers to have fresh open air and feels warm.

NORMAL LABOR

If labor is progressing without a hitch, there is no need to use the labor remedies. *Arnica montana* is the only homeopathic medicine that I use routinely during childbirth. Take *Arnica* 30C *or* 200C (200C is preferable) at the beginning of labor, and repeat hourly until birth. Use 3 to 4 times per day following delivery for a few days. Most practitioners also give one dose of *Caulophyllum*. With homeopathic medicines there is no contraindication if a cesarean section (surgery) is needed.

EXTREME LABOR PAINS

Every labor presents with a certain amount of expected discomfort, however the following list of homeopathic medicines are indicated for labor pains that are excessive and extreme in nature. A well-chosen remedy will bring calm, and allow her to tolerate labor.

✿ *Aconitum napellus* is indicated for extreme labor pains stemming from fear and anxiety. Panic-stricken and tense, she feels as if she could die (although this is not usually the case). She has difficulty breathing through the contractions which come on rapidly, overwhelming her.

✿ *Chamomilla* is a well-known remedy for colicky, fussy babies. It is also indicated for mothers in labor who are hypersensitive to the pains, out of proportion to the contraction itself. She may appear childish, with tantrums, lashing out at her husband (and practitioner). As midwife and homeopath Sandra Perko writes in her book for practitioners, "*Chamomilla* is not a pleasant lady at labor time. If she were an animal, she would bite someone!... *Chamomilla* is known as the seven Fs remedy: fretful, frantic, fussy, finicky, frenzied, furious, and fault-finding." Ouch!

✿ *Nux vomica* is indicated for severe labor pains that may cause fainting (see *Pulsatilla* and *Cimicifuga*). Consider *Nux vomica* when a woman complains of wanting to defecate or urinate but is unable to do so. She is also irritable, angry, and impatient. *Nux vomica* is often indicated for adults who are type A personality and drink a lot of coffee and alcohol.

✿ *Sepia* is for extreme pain associated with a violent bearing-down sensation, as if everything will come out of her womb. *Sepia* is also indicated for women who feel detached, and may have not wanted to be pregnant. Her mood can be irritable and sad.

DIFFICULT, SLOW LABOR: FAILURE TO PROGRESS

Every labor is unique. Some labors have a difficult time "getting off the ground," while others begin easily, contractions are regular, and all of a sudden everything slows down. There can be many reasons why a labor would become dysfunctional, irregular, or slow. With a multitude of variances, our labors do not necessarily follow the textbooks. Possible causes could be due to the cervix not dilating, one's emotional state, baby's position, side effects of interventions and medications, and inadequate labor contractions. Sometimes, the practitioner and/or patient are impatient, and failure to progress is really just failure to be patient. The following is a list of homeopathic medicines useful in treating this condition. Dosage can be 30C or 200C every 15 to 30 minutes if needed.

✿ *Caulophyllum* is considered to be useful at the beginning of labor, as it tends to work best early on. Contractions may be weak, but sharp and spasmodic. Contractions may be felt low in the pelvis, where they are less effective. After labor has begun and is well established, *Cimicifuga* can be helpful for complete dilation.

✿ *Cimicifuga* is for labor pains that are felt in the thighs and hips instead of in the uterus. Her mood can be hysterical and pessimistic.

✿ *Gelsemium* is indicated for labor that has already been ongoing for hours, yet there is no significant progress. The cervix has not dilated and is hard, thick, and tight. She feels exhausted, trembles and has muscle aches. The keynote for *Gelsemium* is sleepy and weak during labor.

✿ *Kali carbonicum* is well known for its treatment of back labor, which refers to feeling intense pain in the back during labor which can continue in between contractions. A common cause of back labor is baby's malposition such as occiput posterior. This is also known as sunny-side up (face up), in which baby is facing mothers abdomen instead of her back, causing baby's head to press on her tailbone. Indications for *Kali carb* include feeling that her back is broken. She can also feel chilly and sluggish.

❁ *Pulsatilla* is another common labor remedy for when labor pains are irregular, and she may feel faint. Typical *Pulsatilla* keynotes include feeling emotional and too warm. She feels better with attention, reassurance, and cool fresh air.

AFTERPAINS

After my second birth, I learned about afterpains: those lingering uterine contractions lasting for several days after delivery. Following birth, the uterus contracts to help shrink it to its pre-pregnancy size, and also to prevent excessive bleeding. Discomfort can range from menstrual cramps to labor pains. They are stronger with successive deliveries. I remember doing my labor breathing exercises when the contractions came, which usually occurred while breastfeeding. Although I knew they were normal, I reached for my homeopathic labor medicines, which I found extremely helpful.

❁ *Arnica montana* can be given following delivery, and may help with preventing or minimizing afterpains. Especially indicated for bruised feeling and muscle soreness with difficult births. *Bellis perennis* is similar to *Arnica,* and can be used as a second choice.

❁ *Caulophyllum* is indicated for prolonged labors. The pains are sharp and felt in the lower abdomen. Several doses of *Caulophyllum* completely alleviated my labor-like afterpains.

❁ *Chamomilla* is used for intensely painful afterpains which are intolerable. She is overly sensitive to the pains.

❁ *Cimicifuga* is also for intense afterpains. These contractions are felt in the lower pelvic area and groin. Her mood is pessimistic and gloomy.

❁ *Sepia* can be used for afterpains with a heaviness or lump sensation in the anus. Typical of this remedy profile, there can also be a bearing-down feeling that "as if all would come out of the vagina."

MISCARRIAGE

See "Grief and Sorrow" on page 140

According to American Congress of Obstetricians and Gynecologist (ACOG) 10 to 25 percent of clinically recognized pregnancies will end in miscarriage, usually during the first 13 weeks. For many women, a miscarriage can be difficult and may affect her on physical, mental, and emotional levels. Signs of a miscarriage include back pain, weight loss, painful regular contractions, discharge of pink-tinged mucus to bright bleeding, and passage of tissues and blood clots.

Conventional Treatment

Interventions such as D&C (surgical dilatation and curettage) are used to remove any remaining tissue and reduce the risk of bleeding and infection. In general, the earlier the miscarriage, the more likely the body will be able to pass the embryo without intervention.

Homeopathic Medicines

When possible, many women prefer to try a more natural approach that will not require medical interventions. If you observe signs of a miscarriage, contact your healthcare provider. If a miscarriage has been confirmed, consider the following homeopathic medicines:

- *Arnica* is indicated when she feels the baby is laid crosswise in the uterus. Discharge of continuous, profuse bright red, or coagulated blood. It is used for any complaint, including miscarriage, following a fall, shock, or bruise.

- *Caulophyllum* is used for severe pain in back and sides. Painful contractions in the lower pelvis during miscarriage with slight bleeding, and spasmodic bearing-down sensation. She can be shaky, weak, and exhausted.

- *Cimicifuga* is indicated for miscarriage when painful contractions are accompanied with intense gloomy, dark moods. Miscarriage can be recurrent. Pains fly across abdomen from side to side, causing her to double over in pain. Miscarriage following frightening event, e.g., an accident.

- ✿ *Gelsemium* is used when there are sharp distressing pains moving upward and/or toward the back. She can have muscle aches, and be sleepy and confused.
- ✿ *Ignatia* is a well-known medicine for grief and sobbing, following miscarriage.
- ✿ *Pulsatilla* is for contractions with intermittent passage of black blood, which can be alternating with bright-red gushes. She is warm-blooded, worse in the heat, and weepy.
- ✿ *Sepia* is indicated for miscarriage from the 5th to 7th months. There can be flushes of heat with faintness. She can have a bearing-down sensation with a ball sensation in the rectum.

RETAINED PLACENTA

The third stage of labor following baby's birth is delivery of the placenta in which the uterus gently contracts to expel. Once it is expelled, the healthcare provider will examine the placenta to make sure it is complete, and that there are no remaining parts left in the womb. On rare occasions, the placenta is not pushed out, either partially or in its entirety; this is known as *retained placenta*.

- ✿ *Caulophyllum* is for retained placenta due to a uterus which lacks the strength to expel placenta. She may have partial separation of the placenta. The contractions are ineffective, and she feels weak and exhausted.
- ✿ *Cimicifuga* is indicated for retained placenta with characteristic painful contractions and dark mood.
- ✿ *Pulsatilla* is for retained placenta with intermittent flow of blood. She is weepy and desires cool open air.
- ✿ *Sepia* is used when there are no specific symptoms. She may have sharp shooting pains with a bearing-down sensation. She can feel detached and irritable.

POSTPARTUM WOUND CARE

From a vaginal birth to cesarean section, I use homeopathic medicines in the postpartum period to speed healing. Most of my patients report that homeopathy shortens the healing time and there is less need for prescribed pain medications. Epidurals are puncture wounds, while significant perineal tears and cesarean section (which is a major operation) require sutures. In addition, there can be significant swelling, bruising, and soreness following an uneventful vaginal delivery.

Care and Treatment
Conventional Treatment Following Delivery
The type of postpartum treatments are dependent upon the birth. Following cesarean section or extensive tears, patients are prescribed pain medications and sometimes antibiotics to prevent infection.

Home Treatment
- Rest (see "Forty Day Period" in Chapter 4)
- Use a hot water bottle on the belly as needed.
- Apply ice packs to the perineum when needed.
- Place homemade frozen postpartum care pads on the perineum. These are a must! Make them ahead of time using maxi pads infused with various herbs including witch-hazel, comfrey, lavender, aloe vera gel, and more. Wrap and freeze. Look online or speak to your healthcare provider for more information.
- Herbal sitz bath, compresses, and peri bottle (plastic squirt bottle) are soothing. A sitz bath can be done in the bathtub or by using a large basin and can offer relief for discomfort in the lower part of the body (including delivery, stitches, as well as hemorrhoids, and fissures).
- Apply witch-hazel pads on the perineum.
- Use a peri bottle full of water (or an herbal solution) to soothe the perineal area during and after urination.
- Place your legs up on a stool during bowel movements to minimize straining.
- Spread perineal healing salves on a sanitary napkin.
- Use a doughnut cushion when sitting (for extensive tears and stitches).

Homeopathic Medicines

The following list represents some of the commonly used homeopathic medicines for wound healing. It is best to have the chosen remedies on hand ahead of time so that they can be used immediately following birth. Unlike some herbs and medications, there are no contraindications for using homeopathic medicines right after surgery. A correctly chosen remedy can help with pain relief, speed healing, and may help avoid infection.

Except for *Arnica*, all of these medicines can be taken at a 30C strength. Take at least three times per day. Upon improvement, taper and then discontinue use. Major surgery may require that the remedy be used for several more days. At the first consult with a newborn and family, most of the new mothers in my practice take homeopathic medicines for healing. Trust me, even if there are no stitches, tears, or lacerations, all women experience soreness and appreciate the effectiveness of the remedies.

- ❀ *Arnica montana* is the first medicine to use following any trauma, including bruising and soreness following birth. Consider using *Arnica* after chorionic villus sampling (CVS), amniocentesis, epidural injection, cesarean section, episiotomy, or vaginal tears during delivery. I prescribe *Arnica* 30C (or a higher dose of 200C for severe soreness and surgery) routinely following birth. Homeopaths also treat past injuries with *Arnica* to begin the healing of old wounds, including complaints dating back to a cesarean section. For chronic conditions, consult with a homeopath. *Arnica* is also available topically (e.g., cream, gel, ointment, oil) but should not be used on open wounds.

- ❀ *Bellis perennis* is used for post-operative pain and bruising, especially of deeper tissues such as the abdomen and pelvis. For example, if *Arnica* is not providing significant relief following a cesarean section, try *Bellis*.

- ❀ *Calendula officinalis* (marigold) has antiseptic, astringent, and anti-microbial properties. It relieves pain and speeds the healing of lacerations and open wounds including perineal tears and episiotomies. It is available as a cream, tincture, spray, or ointment. To use a *Calendula* tincture, dilute 1:4 dilution with water and apply to affected area. It can be added to a sitz bath and compress.

❉ *Gelsemium* can be used for anticipation and anxiety, before a procedure or labor.

❉ *Hypericum perforatum* is excellent for injury to nerves, especially in the fingers, toes, nails, tailbone and spinal cord. The characteristic pains are shooting and sharp, and very sensitive to the touch. *Hypericum* is also indicated for puncture wounds following CVS, amniocentesis, and epidural spinal anesthesia.

❉ *Ledum palustre* is also recommended for puncture wounds with much swelling and inflammation, particularly when the inflamed area looks purple, puffy, and is cold to the touch. Similar to *Hypericum, Ledum* can be used following CVS, amniocentesis, and epidural spinal anesthesia.

❉ *Phosphorus* can be used to treat the ill effects from anesthesia and is indicated for nausea and vomiting. She may be fearful and prefer to have company around. There is a craving for cold drinks or ice chips.

❉ *Pyrogenium* is for infection during the postpartum period when vaginal discharge is foul smelling. Known as puerperal fever (or childbed fever), it can include aching and restlessness with fever and chills. Following delivery (including miscarriage and abortion), mother's body is susceptible to infection from the opening of the uterus, retained placenta, and wounds of the perineum and from cesarean section. Although rare nowadays, infection following childbirth used to be of grave concern. For signs of infection, contact your healthcare provider.

❉ *Staphysagria* is useful for surgical wounds and lacerated tissues requiring stitches, including vaginal tears in delivery, episiotomy, and cesarean section.

Natural Medicine Chest

WHEN POSSIBLE, I PREFER natural medicine and treatments for complaints and conditions during pregnancy. In this section, I have listed some of the more commonly used homeopathic medicines for pregnancy and childbirth. Each medicine is presented with an in-depth description, including keynotes or the characteristic symptoms that can help you choose the right remedy (see "Using Homeopathic Medicines" on page 121).

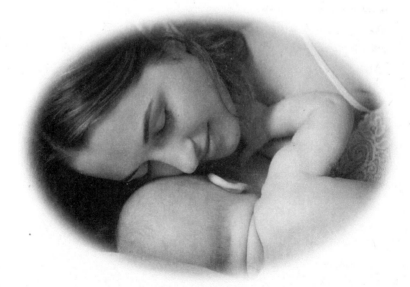

Guide to Homeopathic Medicines (Materia Medica)

ACONITUM NAPELLUS (MONKSHOOD)

Aconitum napellus (Aconite) is also known as SOS, and is truly a rescue medication for a variety of symptoms. It is useful in the treatment in labor when complaints begin very suddenly. *Aconite* can be used for both women and their families when there is a feeling of panic during labor. Consider *Aconite* when there is feeling of shock following an unexpected result from a routine prenatal test.

In January 1994, all of Los Angeles was abruptly awakened to the jolting of a very strong earthquake. Our own house was in complete disarray, but my husband quickly managed to find our homeopathic remedies in the dark. *Aconite* immediately helped calm our shaken nerves. During the week that followed, all the local pharmacies and health food stores claimed to have sold out of this remedy.

***Aconitum napellus* is useful for:**

Mind/Emotions:
- ❀ Anxiety and panic from accidents and frightening or shocking events
- ❀ Feelings of agitation, anxiety, and restlessness
- ❀ Forebodings and fear one will soon die
- ❀ Fear of crowds
- ❀ Claustrophobia
- ❀ Startling easily
- ❀ Sleeplessness and restlessness, with crying and complaining
- ❀ Nightmares and anxious dreams

Body:

- ❀ Sudden onset of intense violent labor pains with feelings of panic and fright
- ❀ Sudden onset palpitations, fevers (excellent medicine in childhood)
- ❀ Intense labor pains that come on suddenly
- ❀ Intolerable labor pains
- ❀ Complaints begin from becoming sweaty and chilled in dry, cold, windy weather
- ❀ Profuse sweating during sleep
- ❀ Chilly if uncovered
- ❀ Face is red, hot, and flushed. One cheek red, the other pale
- ❀ Unquenchable thirst for cold drinks
- ❀ Pulse is full and strong

Symptoms improve with: fresh air, company

Symptoms worsen: at night and evening, in a warm room, lying on affected side, and with noise and light

ARNICA MONTANA (LEOPARD'S BANE)

Arnica is a plant that grows high up in mountain slopes where one could easily get injured in the steep terrain. Hence, *Arnica* is an excellent treatment for trauma. *Arnica* has no contraindications, and is safe for newborns who are bruised, and nursing mothers.

My second labor progressed quickly and my son, Quentin, was born within 3 hours. Although, no specific homeopathic medicine was indicated, I took *Arnica* to help prevent or minimize soreness, bruising, and swelling that happens during birth. It is the only homeopathic medicine that I use routinely during childbirth. Take *Arnica* 200C at the beginning of labor, and repeat hourly until birth. Use three to four times per day following delivery, for a few days. There is no contraindication if a cesarean section (surgery) is needed.

After all is said and done, keep *Arnica* (low potency from 6C to 30C) in your diaper bag.

Arnica montana is useful for:

Mind/Emotions:
- ✿ Restlessness
- ✿ When bed and chairs feel too hard
- ✿ When constantly changing position
- ✿ When says there is nothing wrong, despite being in pain
- ✿ When desire to be alone
- ✿ Irritableness
- ✿ Shock, trauma following an injury or emergency cesarean section

Body:
- ✿ Bruises, swelling, and muscle soreness
- ✿ Body feels "beaten up"
- ✿ Bruised sensation in any part of the body
- ✿ Sprains, strains, and concussions
- ✿ Injuries and bleeding from trauma and accidents
- ✿ After-surgery swelling (caesarean section)

Labor:
- ✿ Any complaint following fall, shock, or bruise
- ✿ Premature labor following an injury, accident or overuse
- ✿ Violent labor pains with soreness in the back
- ✿ Retained placenta
- ✿ Prevention of afterpains if given at the end of labor, indicated for violent pains excited by breastfeeding
- ✿ Muscle soreness following a prolonged difficult labor (see *Bellis perennis*)
- ✿ Baby: use for any bruises, including head bruises from difficult labor

Symptoms improve: when left alone, lying down, outstretched or with the head low

Symptoms worsen: with touch, when jarred, or with cold and damp weather

CAULOPHYLLUM THALICTROIDES
(BLUE COHOSH)

Caulophyllum is well known as a remedy for childbirth, as its primary action is on the uterus. Used for labor in the early stages, it is especially helpful when labor has stalled, and pains are irregular. Indigenous to the United States and Canada, Native Americans considered *Caulophyllum* as their most valuable medicine in labor. It was given to pregnant women as a tea made from an infusion of the root for a few weeks before labor, "Rendering delivery rapid and comparatively painless." (Charles Millspaugh M.D., 19th century). This has been used for generations among homeopaths with great success.

Many practitioners prescribe *Caulophyllum* (sometimes even one dose during labor) with pregnant patients as it is known to regulate and keep pregnancy and labor normal. Caution: Use *Caulophyllum* only at the end of pregnancy as it can induce contractions, yet it is also used to premature labor.

Both *Caulophyllum* and *Cimicifuga* have been a staple in homeopathic practitioners' birth kits. I used Caulophyllum not only for my early labors but for joint pain. At the end of my pregnancies, it was difficult to walk barefoot in the morning because my feet ached. Also, I learned about afterpains following my second birth. A couple of doses of *Caulophyllum* completely alleviated my discomfort.

Caulophyllum is useful for:

Mind/Emotions:
- Nervous and excitable
- Hysterical
- Changeable moods during labor

Body:
- Weakness and exhausted
- Joint pain (rheumatism) of the fingers and toes
- Trembling
- Thirsty

Labor:

- ✿ Dysfunctional labor
- ✿ Sharp, cramp-like intermittent pains
- ✿ Pains moving to the thighs, into groin and bladder
- ✿ Painful spasms in the lower segment of the uterus which are felt in all directions
- ✿ No progress or dilation
- ✿ Cervix remains rigid and tightly closed
- ✿ Difficult and prolonged labors that get "stuck"
- ✿ Miscarriage with severe pain in back and sides. Painful contractions with slight bleeding and spasmodic bearing-down sensation
- ✿ Premature labor, prevention due to weak cervix
- ✿ Kicks-start a genuine labor from a difficult, false one
- ✿ Retained placenta due to a uterus which lacks the strength to expel placenta
- ✿ Bleeding in the postpartum period that is profuse or oozing following a hasty labor
- ✿ Bloody discharge that continues long after birth
- ✿ Afterpains felt low down with bearing-down sensation. Sometimes extends into the groins

Symptoms improve: with warmth

Symptoms worsen: with cold, open air, motion

CIMICIFUGA RACEMOSA (BLACK COHOSH)

Cimicifuga, also a woman's remedy, is well known for treatment of pain affecting both nerves and muscles, including neck, back, and uterus. An indigenous plant in North America, it is known by the Native Americans as squawroot, and is used to facilitate labor. Many of the complaints resemble those treated by *Caulophyllum*; however *Cimicifuga* is recognized by the intense, gloomy dark mood. Many times practitioners have been known to use both remedies during labor.

Cimicifuga is useful for:

Mind/Emotions:
- ❀ Gloom and doom mood
- ❀ Feeling of a dark cloud over everything
- ❀ Pessimistic outlook
- ❀ Extroverted, chatty, and excitable
- ❀ Hysterical with pains
- ❀ Intolerant of the pains
- ❀ Fearful with many phobias
- ❀ Feeling she is going crazy
- ❀ Says "I can't do this." "I can't go through labor."
- ❀ Frequent sighing
- ❀ Premonition that something bad will happen
- ❀ History of difficult past labor, miscarriage, abortion

Body:
- ❀ Sharp muscle pain
- ❀ Neck and back spasm and stiffness
- ❀ Spinal injury
- ❀ Shivering
- ❀ Joint pain (rheumatism)
- ❀ Headaches with muscle stiffness
- ❀ Painful periods, postpartum depression, and infertility

Labor:
- ❀ Dysfunctional labor that stalls
- ❀ Contractions are strong, painful, yet the labor fails to progress
- ❀ Cervix remains rigid despite painful contractions
- ❀ Shooting pains across the pelvis from hip to hip, or into thighs with nervous agitation
- ❀ Spasms, sharp pains, electric shocks, across the belly
- ❀ Doubled over in pain, and crying out
- ❀ Recurrent miscarriage

- ✿ Pains fly across abdomen from side to side, causing her to double over in pain
- ✿ Miscarriage following frightening event, e.g., accident
- ✿ Premature labor
- ✿ False labor
- ✿ Retained placenta
- ✿ Afterpains
- ✿ Postpartum hemorrhage, dark, with clots

Symptoms improve: with warmth, open air, motion, pressure, grasping things, rest, eating

Symptoms worsen: with damp, cold air, change of weather, motion

GELSEMIUM (YELLOW JASMINE)

Gelsemium is well known as a flu remedy, with weakness as the particular keynote symptom. In addition, this remedy is called for when someone lacks confidence before facing a challenge—such as labor and delivery. The symptoms of weakness, anxiety, and trembling all point to *Gelsemium*. With complaints of fatigue and nervousness, it can be used when *Caulophyllum* fails to work.

At the end of my labor when I was getting more tired and running out of steam, my midwife gave me a dose of *Gelsemium* which helped my labor progress smoothly until the end.

Gelsemium **is useful for:**

Mind/Emotions:
- ✿ Fearful and frightened easily
- ✿ Anticipatory anxiety before due date
- ✿ Performance anxiety if too many people present at labor
- ✿ Cowardice

❀ Trembling
❀ Sleepy, dull, and apathetic
❀ For men who feel faint during birth

Body:

❀ Flu-like ache
❀ Great fatigue and exhaustion
❀ Extreme weakness
❀ Heaviness of eyelids, limbs, and body
❀ Dizziness, muscle aches, and trembling in labor
❀ Difficulty sleeping from excitement and worry

Labor:

❀ Miscarriage with sharp distressing pains moving upward and/or toward the back
❀ Confused feeling
❀ Dysfunctional labor
❀ Failure to dilate and progress
❀ False labor pains
❀ Failure to progress
❀ Cervix is rigid, thick
❀ Pains felt upward and to the back
❀ Severe, sharp pains extending to the back and hips
❀ Labor ceases at end of labor even though fully dilated
❀ Retained placenta with pains in lower abdomen moving upwards and backward
❀ Afterpains with pains running upward and/or toward the back
❀ Pains lasting too long with muscular weakness

Symptoms improve in the afternoon and with: cold, open air, urination, sweating, bending forward, lying down with head propped up

Symptoms worsen: with motion, damp weather, excitement, at about 10 a.m.

IGNATIA AMARA
(ST. IGNATIUS BEAN)

Ignatia is a well-known remedy for emotional upheavals, including grief, loss, and sorrow. A few doses of *Ignatia* were extremely helpful for my teary moments that came from the wave of hormonal changes in the first weeks of becoming a mom. Consider *Ignatia* for a woman who is greatly disappointed with a sense of grief that her birth did not proceed as planned (e.g., unexpected use of interventions, cesarean section, etc.).

Ignatia is useful for:

Mind/Emotions:
- Tendency toward sobbing, sadness, and sighing
- Frequent yawning
- Aversion to being consoled
- Hysterical symptoms
- Oversensitive and anxious
- Alternating moods (hysterical crying to laughing)
- Labor and miscarriage with accompanying grief
- Postpartum depression
- Stillbirth

Body:
- Physical complaints originating from disappointment, grief, sorrow
- Difficulty nursing
- Lump in the throat
- Numbness, twitches, and spasms
- Craving for cheese

Labor:
- Miscarriage, labor, afterpains, etc., with characteristic emotional symptoms of sobbing, hysteria, despondency, and sighing

Symptoms improve: with eating, change of position, being alone, deep breathing

Symptoms worsen: with cold, touch, coffee

KALI CARBONICUM (POTASSIUM CARBONATE)

Kali carbonicum is used for back labor often associated with a baby who is positioned posterior (sunny-side-up) instead of the optimal anterior position with baby's back to mother's belly. With my first birth, my son was born sunny-side-up. Although I did not experience back labor, I kept this remedy nearby in case I needed it for the next one.

One of my patients, who was 9 months pregnant, was seen for a nagging stitching pain in the lower belly. She had to hold her belly when moving and with bending. After one dose of *Kali carbonicum* 200C, her pain subsided and did not return. She went on to deliver a healthy boy several weeks later.

Kali carbonicum is useful for:

Mind/Emotions:
- ✿ Worry about practical matters (baby, finance, etc)

Body:
- ✿ Chilly
- ✿ Trembling
- ✿ Belching
- ✿ Stitching pains (side ache or cramp)
- ✿ Painful cough, worse at 2 to 4 a.m.

Labor:
- ✿ Back labor
- ✿ Severe back pains, as if "back will break"
- ✿ Back pains that extend down to buttock muscles
- ✿ Postpartum hemorrhage with back pain

Symptoms improve: with pressure on back, back rubbed, warm weather

Symptoms worsen: when sensitive to cold, at 2 to 4 a.m.

NATRUM MURIATICUM (COMMON SALT)

Natrum muriaticum is a well-known remedy for grief. It is indicated for many conditions in pregnancy and labor, especially when there is a component of melancholy, sadness, and suffering (including from past experiences). It is reminiscent of our salty tears.

***Natrum muriaticum* is useful for:**

Mind/Emotions:
- ✿ Grief, loss, unrequited love
- ✿ Loneliness
- ✿ Sensitive, easily hurt feelings
- ✿ Averse to company and consolation
- ✿ Desire for solitude
- ✿ Desire to cry when alone (but may be unable to cry)

Body:
- ✿ Labor progresses slowly with weak contractions
- ✿ Dryness of mouth, throat, nose
- ✿ Dry, cracked lips (center lower lip)
- ✿ Allergies, stuffy nose with egg white–like discharge
- ✿ Headaches, worse from sun, heat, light, noise, study
- ✿ Cold sores and herpes outbreak
- ✿ Thirsty for cold drinks
- ✿ Craving for salty foods, lemon, and chocolate

Symptoms improve: with fresh air

Symptoms worsen: in sun, at about 10 a.m.

NUX VOMICA (QUAKER BUTTONS)

Nux vomica is an excellent remedy for "too much"—too much work, food, drink, and stress. But its powers extend beyond relieving indigestion after a Thanksgiving meal; it can also be used for labor pains and conditions in pregnancy including colds, constipation, heartburn, hemorrhoids, and the kind of insomnia brought on by doing—you guessed it—too much.

Nux vomica is useful for:

Mind/Emotions:
- ❀ Hardworking personality (Type A)
- ❀ Competitive
- ❀ Irritable, impatient, and angry
- ❀ Easily frustrated

Body:
- ❀ Spasmodic labor pains with desire for stool
- ❀ Fainting after pains
- ❀ Overeating (especially spicy or rich foods)
- ❀ Weakness from drinking too much coffee
- ❀ Fullness, heartburn, indigestion, upset stomach, vomiting, bloating, and gas
- ❀ Constipation, straining with incomplete sensation
- ❀ Insomnia (from doing too much)
- ❀ Stuffed nose with watery discharge and sneezing, plugged at night, runny during the day
- ❀ Extremely chilly
- ❀ Sensitive to stimuli (noise and light)
- ❀ Difficult sleeping, waking at 3 or 4 a.m.

Symptoms improve: with rest, in the evening

Symptoms worsen: in cold, dry weather, wind, in the early morning, outdoors

PULSATILLA
(PASQUE FLOWER)

Pulsatilla is rich in its history and medicinal uses. The pasque flower blooms at Easter and once was used to color Easter eggs. Since ancient times, it has been valued for its effectiveness in treating conditions of the eye. According to legend, the flower sprang from the tears of Venus. *Pulsatilla* is a windflower, one that sways in the wind. Hence, the woman who responds to *Pulsatilla* has changeable symptoms. She is easily moved to tears. *Pulsatilla* is also used for many complaints throughout pregnancy and birth. This is a common emotional state at least some time during pregnancy. The woman who responds to *Pulsatilla* needs comfort, reassurance, and consolation. She can be weepy.

Pulsatilla is useful for:

Mind/Emotions:
- ✿ Emotional states
- ✿ Fear and concern for the baby
- ✿ When easily moved to tears and laughter
- ✿ Desire for consolation, sympathy, and affection
- ✿ Timid, gentle, and clingy personality
- ✿ Easily irritated, touchy
- ✿ Fears of being alone and in the dark
- ✿ Restlessness, likes to keep busy

Body:
- ✿ Warm-blooded and worse in the heat
- ✿ Craves ice cream, butter, pastries (despite causing indigestion)
- ✿ Lack of thirst, even though has a dry mouth
- ✿ Stuffy feeling in closed room
- ✿ Fainting during labor
- ✿ Needs fanning or fresh air
- ✿ Painful and irregular periods
- ✿ Inflammation with thick yellow discharge in nose, chest, and vagina
- ✿ Indigestion, heartburn from rich foods
- ✿ Breech presentation
- ✿ Breastfeeding aid

Labor
- ✿ False labor
- ✿ Slow, inactive, weak contractions
- ✿ Dysfunctional labor despite dilated cervix
- ✿ Falls asleep during contractions
- ✿ Changeable pains, from weak to strong
- ✿ Irregular contractions
- ✿ Miscarriage contraction with intermittent passage of black blood, can be alternating with bright-red gushes
- ✿ Premature labor
- ✿ Movement of the fetus is violent and painful
- ✿ Retained placenta with intermittent flow of blood

Symptoms improve: in open air, breezes, slow walks outside, cool and crisp weather, cold applications

Symptoms worsen: when alone, in the heat, in a warm and stuffy room, in the evenings and at night, with greasy, rich foods

SEPIA (CUTTLEFISH INK)

Sepia comes from the ink sac of the cuttlefish and has been used in photography (sepia tone). *Sepia* is a common woman's remedy, when her symptoms are aggravated around her period and pregnancy, ranking it an important homeopathic medicine for hormonal and sexual complaints.

Sepia **is useful for:**

Mind/Emotions:
- ✿ Emotionally detached from family, indifference
- ✿ Conscientious about responsibilities
- ✿ Worn out from caring for everyone
- ✿ Prefers to be alone
- ✿ Irritable, easily offended
- ✿ Wants to escape, get away from it all
- ✿ Dragging and sagging

Body:

✿ Lacks energy
✿ Feels better with vigorous exercise
✿ Premenstrual syndrome (PMS), genital herpes
✿ Sagging feeling (face, belly, breasts, etc.)
✿ Prolapse of uterus, bladder with bearing-down sensation
✿ Morning sickness, hemorrhoid, varicose veins, constipation, genital herpes
✿ Faint feeling in pregnancy
✿ Sensation of lump in the rectum
✿ Spots and pigment changes on the face (chloasma, mask of pregnancy)
✿ Craves vinegar, sour food, sweets

Labor:

✿ Miscarriage between 5th and 7th months
✿ Flushes of heat with faintness
✿ Distressing, spasmodic pains
✿ False labor pains
✿ Weight or heavy ball feeling in the anus with constipation
✿ Postpartum bleeding with sensation of weight
✿ Congestion of uterus with sensation of weight, as if all would come out of vagina
✿ Retained placenta with little, sharp shooting pains.
✿ Afterpains with sense of weight in the anus, or bearing down

Symptoms improve: with vigorous exercise, warmth of bed, hot applications, sleep, cold drinks, open air

Symptoms worsen: before period, pregnancy, miscarriage, morning, late afternoon, sex, kneeling, stooping, washing clothes.

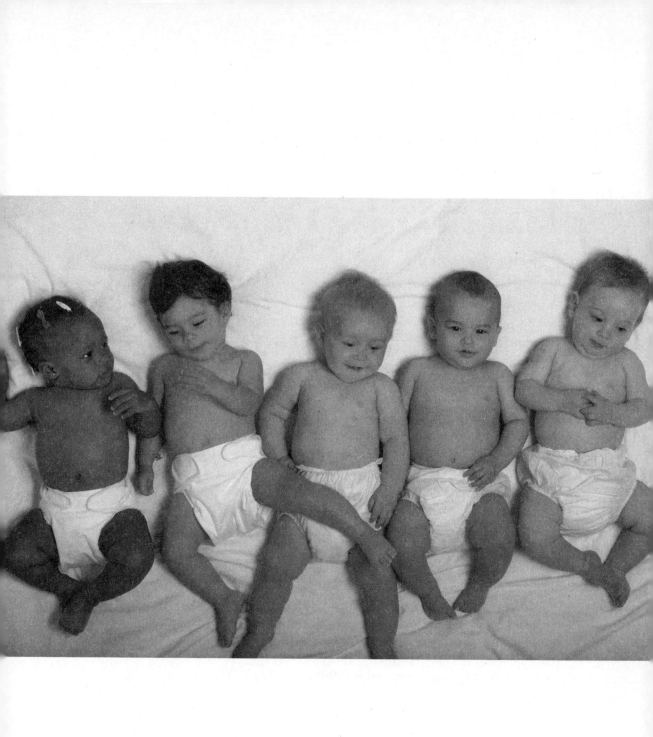

Natural Essentials

I N ADDITION TO HOMEOPATHIC medicines, I have compiled a list of additional remedies, exercises, and natural essentials that are used frequently during pregnancy (and beyond):

Prenatal Vitamins

The more natural brands are usually preferable over the standard prescription ones. A prenatal vitamin is meant to supplement a healthy diet, not replace it. It is best to take vitamins in divided doses throughout the day. (See "Nutrition and Pregnancy" in Chapter 1.)

Red Raspberry Leaf Tea

Red Raspberry Leaf tea is known for toning the muscles of the uterus and the pelvic region. It has been used by pregnant women in the second half of pregnancy for generations. Red raspberry leaves are rich in vitamins and minerals including Vitamin B complex, calcium, iron, and magnesium. It is used for morning sickness, improved circulation, preparing the uterus for an easier birth, and improving milk supply. Drink at least one cup per day in the third trimester.

Placenta Encapsulation

In the womb, the placenta is attached to the wall of the uterus and develops with the baby until they are separated at birth. They are connected through the umbilical cord which arises from it. The placenta provides oxygen, vitamins, and nutrients to the growing baby, and also removes waste products from baby's blood—all via the cord. Normally, the placenta attaches at the top or side of the uterus, but on occasion there are problems including placental abruption (when the placenta peels away from the wall of the uterus), placenta previa (which covers the cervix partially or totally), and placenta accreta (when the blood vessels of the placenta grow too deeply into the uterine wall). All of these can lead to heavy vaginal bleeding. The third stage of labor following baby's birth is delivery of the placenta in which the uterus gently contracts to expel it. Once it is expelled, the healthcare provider will examine it to make sure it is complete, and that there are no remaining parts left in the womb. On rare occasions, the placenta has difficulty being expelled either partially or in its entirety, this is known as *retained placenta* (see "Homeopathy for Childbirth" on page 160).

Many family members (including older siblings) appreciate seeing the placenta which is usually placed in a designated bowl. Many cultures use the placenta in various ways. In our home, we placed it in the freezer and when our babies were a few months old, we buried the placenta to offer new life in the garden. Some women consume the placenta: cooking, eating and encapsulating it, known as human placentophagy.

FROM THE DOCTOR'S DESK

Following a home birth with a moderate amount of postpartum bleeding, Mary was told that she would benefit from eating her placenta to replenish the loss. A devout vegetarian, but fearful that she was too anemic, she consumed her placenta (smoothie style) in the few days postpartum and began to feel more strength and energy. Thereafter, her postpartum period and breastfeeding went smoothly.

For some, eating the afterbirth is a new way of thinking. Humans are one of the only mammals that do not regularly consume the placenta (afterbirth) which is rich in iron, vitamin B_{12}, and hormones. Some ancient cultures ate the placenta, and in Chinese medicine the placenta is prepared and consumed to overcome exhaustion, anemia and other sexual complaints in both women and men. Nowadays, encapsulation is a common method in which the placenta is steamed, dehydrated and pulverized before being placed into capsules. Other women consume it raw in a smoothie or cook it with onion, like liver.

At least half of all the new mothers in my practice use placenta encapsulation and report benefits that improve baby blues, stabilize hormones, increase energy, provide extra iron, stimulate milk production, and speed recovery following delivery. The dosage varies per practitioner (1 to 2 capsules twice per day for 2 to 3 weeks). Because some women complain that they feel "wired" following a dose, it is best to begin slowly with 1 capsule at a time and increase as needed.

Birth Ball

The birth ball can be used during pregnancy and delivery and for soothing a crying baby. For exercise it can help strengthen your core, and it helps with alignment. The rocking pelvic motion can bring relief for back pain and contractions, and facilitates optimal positions for labor. The birth ball is versatile and has a myriad of functions. Some women bring their ball to their birthplace. You can even ask to be monitored (through electronic fetal monitoring) while sitting on the ball.

Hot Water Bottle

Used by our grandparents and their parents before them, the hot water bottle is an essential part of every family's medicine chest. As a symbol of warmth and security, its uses vary from warming up a cold bed to soothing cramps and comforting mental anguish. To avoid burns, follow the manufacturer's instructions when using. While holding the neck of the bottle, carefully pour the hot water up to half full. Expel remaining air by folding over the empty top half, and screw cap tightly. Wrap with a soft protective cloth before use. This can be used for cramps, soreness, and chills.

Kegel Exercises

Kegels are pelvic floor strengthening exercises. During pregnancy and especially following delivery, women are susceptible to weakening of these muscles which can lead to urinary incontinence and pelvic organ prolapse. A strong pelvic floor supports the uterus, bladder, and bowels. The Kegel technique is performed by intentionally contracting the muscles of the pelvic floor. Be sure to relax fully after each contraction. It is advisable to do at least 25 daily on a regular schedule, now and in the years to come.

Labor At-A-Glance

COMMON SYMPTOMS	NATURAL TREATMENTS AND HOMEOPATHY
General and Normal Labor	Change position every 45 minutes. Eat lightly as desired. Drink frequently. Urinate every hour. Avoid IVs when possible (use hep-lock if needed). Homeopathic medicines: *Arnica* (use hourly during labor), *Caulophyllum* (give one dose). See "Comfort Measures During Labor" (page 74) and "Tips on Having a Natural Undisturbed Birth" (page 81).
Overdue: Natural Approach to Induce Labor	Have sex. Stimulate nipples. Walk. Try Castor oil and Evening primrose oil. Eat spicy foods. Drink Raspberry Leaf Tea. Seek holistic treatment: acupressure, chiropractic, etc. Homeopathic medicines: *Arnica, Caulophyllum, Cimicifuga, Gelsemium, Pulsatilla.*
False Labor	Homeopathic medicines: *Caulophyllum* (first choice). *Cimicifuga, Pulsatilla.*
Extreme Labor Pains	Homeopathic medicines: *Aconite, Chamomilla, Nux vomica, Sepia.*
Difficult, Slow Labor: Failure to Progress	Homeopathic medicines: *Caulophyllum* (early labor), *Cimicifuga, Gelsemium* (later in labor), *Kali carbonicum* (back labor), *Pulsatilla.*
Back Labor	Move and change position. Homeopathic medicine: *Kali carbonicum.*
Retained Placenta	Homeopathic medicines: *Caulophyllum, Cimicifuga, Gelsemium, Pulsatilla, Sepia.*
Afterpains	Homeopathic medicines: *Arnica, Caulophyllum, Chamomilla, Cimicifuga, Sepia.*
Nervousness and Anxiety (for mother and others)	Homeopathic medicines: *Aconite, Arsenicum album, Gelsemium, Phosphorus.* Bach Flower Essence: *Rescue Remedy.*

Commonly Used Homeopathic Medicines During Labor

Aconitum napellus (Aconite)	*Sudden and intense complaints:* Feels anxious, agitated and restless. In a panic. Violent and intolerable labor pains. Thirsty for cold drinks. Feels better with fresh air and company.
Arnica montana (Arnica)	*Bruising and muscle soreness:* Use routinely during labor and after birth, including following a cesarean section. Use for baby if bruised.
Caulophyllum	*Difficult stalled labor:* Valuable childbirth remedy. Helpful for many aspects of labor and delivery, especially when not progressing in early labor. Feels sharp pains in lower uterus that move in all directions, including down thigh. Cervix fails to dilate. Trembles, feels weak and exhausted. Can also have joint pain. Use *Caulphyllum* in labor if no other symptoms point to other remedies.
Cimicifuga	*"I can't go through labor":* Important childbirth medicine similar to *Caulophyllum*. Complains of sharp pains, trembling and nervousness. Mood is characteristic: dark, pessimistic, gloom and doom. She is excitable, hysterical and fearful. May have history of difficult past experiences: e.g., miscarriage, abortion.
Gelsemium	*Anticipation and weakness:* For nervous anticipation before due date. Use at end of labor when *Caulophyllum* fails to act. Labor ceases at end, even though fully dilated Feels weak and sleepy.
Pulsatilla	*Emotional with changeable contractions:* For labor with dysfunctional contractions that change from weak to strong. Desires company but easily irritated and moved to tears. Feels warm and prefers fresh air. Also used for breech presentation, indigestion, and breastfeeding.
Sepia	*Worn out and dragging:* Common female medicine, used for distressing labor pains with bearing-down sensation. Feels exhausted, better with exercise. Wants to be left alone. Lump sensation in anus. Also useful for morning sickness, hemorrhoids, and constipation. Craves vinegar and sour foods.

T HE FOLLOWING IS A list of organizations and books or other resources where you can find more information about the topics discussed in this book. In addition, there are some commonly used brands of natural products and homeopathic medicines available on the web, in health food stores, and in homeopathic pharmacies.

www.drfeder.com

DrFeder.com is a content-rich resource on homeopathy, holistic medicine, and natural parenting. The website also features a family of experts in the fields of pregnancy, natural childbirth, naturopathic medicine, nutrition, massage, feng shui, philosophy, and animal health. For your convenience, DrFeder.com also carries a comprehensive line of homeopathic medicines mentioned in this book.

Healthcare Providers and Holistic Practitioners

American College of Nurse-Midwives (ACNM)
www.midwife.org

American Congress of Obstetricians and Gynecologists (ACOG)
www.acog.org

Midwives Alliance of North America (MANA)
www.mana.org

National Center for Homeopathy
www.homeopathic.org

Childbirth Organizations and Natural Parenting Education

Attachment Parenting International
www.attachmentparenting.org

Birthworks International
www.birthworks.org

Bradley Method
www.bradleybirth.com

Childbirth and Postpartum Professional Association (CAPPA)
www.icappa.net

Coalition for Improving Maternity Services (CIMS)/ Mother-Friendly
Childbirth Initiative
www.motherfriendly.org

Doulas of North America (DONA International)
www.dona.org

Holistic Moms Network
www.holisticmoms.org

Hypnobabies
www.hypnobabies.com

International Cesarean Awareness Network (ICAN)
www.ican-online.org

La Leche League International (Breastfeeding)
www.llli.org

Dr. Mercola's Natural Health Information
www.mercola.com

National Vaccine Information Center (NVIC)
www.nvic.org

Spinning Babies
www.spinningbabies.com

Nutrition

Dr. Brewer Pregnancy Diet
www.drbrewerpregnancydiet.com

Weston A. Price Foundation
www.westonaprice.org

Homeopathic Medicines and Bach Flowers

Boiron
www.boiron.com

Hahnemann Laboratories and Pharmacy
(888) 4-ARNICA

Hyland's and Standard Homeopathic Company
www.hylands.com

Nelson Bach USA Ltd (Rescue Remedy and other Bach Flower Essences)
www.nelsonbach.com

Books and DVDs

Beyond the Sling: A Real-Life Guide to Raising Confident, Loving Children the Attachment Parenting Way, by Mayim Bialik. (Touchstone 2012)

The Business of Being Born
www.thebusinessofbeingborn.com

Gentle Birth, Gentle Mothering, by Sarah J. Buckley, M.D. (Celestial Arts 2009).

Happy Healthy Child,—childbirth education DVD series.

Homeopathic Medicines for Pregnancy and Childbirth, by Richard Moskowitz, M.D. (North Atlantic Books. 1992)

Homeopathy for Pregnancy, Birth, and Your Baby's First Year, by Miranda Castro (Macmillan London Ltd. 1993)

Homeopathy for the Modern Pregnant Woman and Her Infant: A Therapeutic Practice Guidebook for Midwives, Physicians and Practitioners, by Sandra J. Perko (Benchmark Homeopathic Publications 1997).

Ina May's Guide to Childbirth, by Ina May Gaskin (Bantam Books, 2003)

Natural Baby and Childcare, by Lauren Feder, M.D. (Hatherleigh Press. 2006)

The Parents' Concise Guide to Childhood Vaccinations, by Lauren Feder, M.D,. (Hatherleigh Press. 2007)

REFERENCES

Introduction to Natural Pregnancy

"Achievements in Public Health, 1900–1999: Healthier Mothers and Babies." *MMWR Weekly.* October 1, 1999/ 48(38); 849–858.
http://www.cdc.gov/mmwr/preview/mmwrhtml/mm4838a2.htm

Unicef Office of Research. *The Decline of Infant Mortality in Europe, 1800–1950: Four national case studies*

Kukla, Rebecca and Wayne, Katherine, "Pregnancy, Birth, and Medicine," *The Stanford Encyclopedia of Philosophy* (Spring 2011 Edition), Edward N. Zalta (ed.).
http://plato.stanford.edu/archives/spr2011/entries/ethics-pregnancy/

Pregnancy, Birth, and Medicine Feb 17, 2011
http://plato.stanford.edu/entries/ethics-pregnancy/#PreDiaScr

Science News. "The Nocebo Effect: Media Reports May Trigger Symptoms of a Disease." May 2013.
http://www.sciencedaily.com/releases/2013/05/130506095305.htm

Lothian, Judith A. RN, PhD, LCCE, FACCE. *J Perinat Educ.*2000. "Why Natural Childbirth"
http://www.ncbi.nlm.nih.gov/pmc/articles/PMC1595040/

"Placebo Effect Works Both Ways: Beliefs About Pain Levels Appear to Override Effects of Potent Pain-Relieving Drug." *Science News.* Feb. 27, 2011.

Wilson, B.L.. "The Influence of Hospitals, Providers and Patients in Birth Outcomes Following Induction of Labor," University of Arizona, College of Nursing. 2008.

Lane, Hilary J., MLS, Nava Blum, PhD, & Elizabeth Fee, PhD. "Oliver Wendell Holmes (1809–1894) and Ignaz Philipp Semmelweis (1818–1865): Preventing the Transmission of Puerperal Fever"
http://www.ncbi.nlm.nih.gov/pmc/articles/PMC2866610/

Chamberlain, Geoffrey. "British maternal mortality in the 19th and early 20th centuries." *J R Soc Med.* 2006 November; 99(11): 559–563. *Journal Royal Society of Medicine.*
http://www.ncbi.nlm.nih.gov/pmc/articles/PMC1633559/

Chapter 1—Optimizing Your Health: Before, During, and After Pregnancy

"Fetus to Mom: You're Stressing Me Out!" MedicineNet.com

spinningbabies.com

Elise L. LeMoyne, Daniel Curnier. "The effects of exercise during pregnancy on the newborn's brain." 2012. Trialsjournal.com

All Exercise is Labor Prep. FitPregnancy.com

University of Sydney at glycemicindex.com.

Weston A. Price Foundation. *Nourishing Traditions*, by Sally Fallon and Mary Enig.

Chapter 2—Making Decisions: Practitioner, Birthplace, and Prenatal Tests

American College of Nurse-Midwives. CNM. www.midwife.org

Midwifery Education Accreditation Council. www.meacschool.org

Janssen, PhD, Patricia A., Saxell, MA, Lee. "Outcomes of planned home birth with registered midwife versus planned hospital birth with midwife or physician." *Canadian Medical Association Journal.* CMAJ. 2009.
http://www.ncbi.nlm.nih.gov/pmc/articles/PMC2742137/

Klaus, M.D. Marshall, & Kennell, M.D. , John. *Mothering the Mother. How A Doula Can Help You Have A Shorter, Easier, And Healthier Birth.* (DaCapo Press 1993).

Trueba, Guadalupe, LCCE, FACCE, CD (DONA). "Alternative Strategy to Decrease Cesarean Section: Support by Doulas During Labor"
http://www.ncbi.nlm.nih.gov/pmc/articles/PMC1595013/

Kieler H., Cnattingius S., Haglund B., Palmgren J., & Axelsson O. "Sinistrality—a side-effect of prenatal sonography: A comparative study of young men." SourceDepartment of Women's and Children's Health, Obstetrics and Gynecology, Uppsala University, Sweden.

McKune, Dorothy. Michel Odent Interview. October 2012.

"Prenatal exposure to ultrasound waves impacts neuronal migration in mice," Proceedings of the National Academy of Sciences, 2006 103: 12903–12910.

Newnham, J.P., Evans, S.F., Michael, C.A., Stanley, F.J., & Landau, L. I. (1993). "Effects of Frequent Ultrasound During Pregnancy: A Randomized Controlled Trial." *The Lancet*, 342(Oct.9), 887–891.

Campbell, J.D., Elford, R.W. & Brant, R.F. (1993). "Case-Controlled Study of Prenatal Ultrasound Exposure in Children with Delayed Speech." *Canadian Medical Association Journal*, 149(10), 1435–1440.

American Congress of Obstetricians and Gynecologists (ACOG). *Ultrasound Exams. Acr–Acog–Aium–Sru Practice Guideline for the Performance of Obstetrical Ultrasound 2013.* Association for Improvements in the Maternity Services.

Woo. Joseph, Dr. "A short History of the development of Ultrasound in Obstetrics and Gynecology." SciLinks. 2002.
http://www.ob-ultrasound.net/history1.html

Beech, Beverley. 1995. "Ultrasound—The Mythology of a Safe and Painless Technology." A Paper presented to the Royal Society of Medicine, October 1995.

Buckley, Sarah. MD. Ultrasound Scans—Cause for Concern. *Gentle Birth, Gentle Mothering,* (Celestial Arts 2009).

"Diagnostic Ultrasound Safety: A summary of the technical report "Exposure Criteria for Medical Diagnostic Ultrasound:II. Criteria Based on all Known Mechanisms," issued by the National Council on Radiation Protection and Measurements.

Salvesen K.A., Vatten L.J., Eik-Nes S.H., Hugdahl K., & Bakketeig L.S. "Routine ultrasonography in utero and subsequent handedness and neurological development." Department of Gynaecology and Obstetrics, University Medical Centre, Trondheim, Norway.

Newnham J.P., Evans S.F., Michael C.A., Stanley F.J., & Landau L.I. "Effects of frequent ultrasound during pregnancy: a randomised controlled trial." *The Lancet*. 1993.

Centers for Disease Control and Prevention. "Group B Strep Fast Facts." 2012. http://www.cdc.gov/groupbstrep/about/fast-facts.html

American Pregnancy Association. "Group B Strep Infection."
http://americanpregnancy.org/pregnancycomplications/groupbstrepinfection.html11.

P.F. Katz et al., "Group B Streptococcus: To Culture or Not to Culture?," *Journal of Perinatology* 19, no. 5 (1999): 37–42.

Noveli, Christa. "Treating Group B Strep: Are Antibiotics Necessary?" *Mothering Magazine.* Nov/Dec 2003.

Bedford Russell AR, Murch SH.. "Could peripartum antibiotics have delayed health consequences for the infant?" *BJOG.* 2006 Jul;113(7):758–65.

Dekker, PhD. Rebecca. "Group B Strep in Pregnancy: Evidence for Antibiotics and Alternatives". Evidence Based Birth.
http://evidencebasedbirth.com/groupbstrep/

Gardner S.E., Yow, M.D., Leeds, L.J., Thompson, P.K., Mason, E.O., Jr, Clark D.J. "PubMedFailure of penicillin to eradicate group B streptococcal colonization in the pregnant woman. A couple study."
http://www.ncbi.nlm.nih.gov/pubmed/391044

Saldana, T.M., Basso, O., Hoppin, J.A., Baird, D.D., Knott, C., Blair, A., Alavanja, M.C., & Sandler, D.P. "Pesticide exposure and self-reported gestational diabetes mellitus in the Agricultural Health Study." *Diabetes Care.* 2007
http://www.ncbi.nlm.nih.gov/pubmed/17327316

Lamar, M.E., Kuehl, T.J., Cooney, A.T., Gayle, L.J., Holleman, S., & Allen S.R. "Jelly beans as an alternative to a fifty-gram glucose beverage for gestational diabetes screening." *Am J Obstet Gynecol.* 1999 Nov;181(5 Pt 1):1154–7.

Jovanovic-Peterson L., & M. Peterson, C.M. "Is exercise safe or useful for gestational diabetic women?" *Diabetes.* 1991 Dec;40 Suppl 2:179–81.

Rhophylac Drug Information. Uptodate.com

Fisher, Barbara Loe. Vaccination During Pregnancy: Is It Safe: National Vaccine Information Center. NVIC. 2013.

Chapter 3—The Wonderment of Childbirth: Natural Birth and the Medical Approach

Lothan, Judith. RN PhD. Do Not Disturb: The Importance of Privacy in Labor. *Journal of Perinatal Education.* 2004.
http://www.oneworldbirth.net/videos/michel-odent-on-the-love-cocktails-in-birth/

Gravotta, Luciana. "Be Mine Forever: Oxytocin May Help Build Long-Lasting Love." *Scientific American.* February 2013.

Korte, Diana. "Birth After Cesarean: A Primer for Success." Issue 89, July/August 1998. http://birthingalternatives.com/Resources/Cesarean/Birth%20After%20 Cesarean.pdf

Hotelling, Barbara, WHNP-BC, CD (DONA), LCCE. "From Psychoprophylactic to Orgasmic Birth." *Journal of Perinatal Education.* 2009. http://www.ncbi.nlm.nih.gov/pmc/articles/PMC2776526/

Comfort Technique. "Vocalization." BirthingNaturally.com

Geiss, Erika-Marie. "Easing Tension and Fear in Natural Childbirth by Understanding Sphincter Law." A Conversation with Ina May Gaskin. 2011.

Birthologie. What you don't know about your cervix can ruin your birth. http://www.birthologie.com/birth/what-you-dont-know-about-your-cervix/

Effacement. American Pregnancy Association

Robin Elise Weiss, LCCE. Labor Station—Your Baby's Position in Relation to the Pelvis. About.com.

Sommers, Anne, & Jones, Carl. "Water Birth." Dear Midwife.com

Water Birth. American Pregnancy Association

Burns E, Blamey C., "The use of aromatherapy in intrapartum midwifery practice an observational study." *Complement Ther Nurs Midwifery.* 2000

Excerpted from "Everything You Need to Know to Prevent Perineal Tearing," by Elizabeth Bruce, *Midwifery Today* Issue 65. The remainder of the article will be excerpted in E-News Issue 6:1

Georgina Stamp. Gillian Kruzins. Perineal massage in labour and prevention of perineal trauma: randomised controlled trial British Medical Journal. *BMJ.* 2001 May 26. http://www.ncbi.nlm.nih.gov/pmc/articles/PMC31922/

ACOG Recommends Restricted Use of Episiotomies. ACOG. 2006

Fogelson, Nicholas. MD. Delayed Cord Clamping. Dept of Obstetrics and Gyneocology. USC School of Medicine.

McDonald, S.J., & Middleton, P. "Effect of timing of umbilical cord clamping of term infants on maternal and neonatal outcomes." Midwifery Professorial Unit, Mercy Hospital for Women, Level 4, Room 4.071, 163 Studley Road, Heidelberg, Victoria, Australia, 2003.

"Delayed Cord Clamping After Birth Better for Baby's Health." *Medical News Today*. 2013.
http://www.medicalnewstoday.com/articles/263181.php

Levy, Karen. "My Baby, My Microbiome Women in the World." Emory University 2013.
http://www.thedailybeast.com/witw/articles/2013/06/02/babies-born-by-cesarean-section-may-not-gain-benefits-of-vaginal-microbiome.html

de Weerth, Carolina,, PhDa., & Susana Fuentes, PhDb. "Intestinal Microbiota of Infants With Colic: Development and Specific Signatures." *Pediatrics* January 14, 2013.

Rebecca L. Dekker, PhD. "Are IV Fluids Necessary during Labor?" Evidence Based Birth. 2012.
http://evidencebasedbirth.com/are-iv-fluids-necessary-during-labor/

Singata, M., Tranmer, J., & Gyte, G.M.L. "Eating and drinking in labour." *Cochrane Summaries*. 2013

Mongeli, M., Wilcox, M., "Estimating the date of confinement: ultrasonographic biometry versus certain menstrual dates." *Am J Obstet Gynecol*. 1996. Department of Obstetrics and Gynaecology, Queen's Medical Centre, Nottingham, United Kingdom.
http://www.ncbi.nlm.nih.gov/pubmed/8572021?dopt=Abstract

Robin Elise Weiss, LCCE. "The Myth of a Vaginal Exam: Why a Vaginal Exam at the End of Pregnancy Might Not Be What You Think." About.com

Phelps, J.Y., Higby, K., Smyth, M.H., Ward, J.A., Arredondo, F., & Mayer A.R. Accuracy and intraobserver variability of simulated cervical dilatation measurements. *Am J Obstet Gynecol*. 1995 Sep;173(3 Pt 1):942–5.

Shephard, A., & Cheyne, H. "The purple line as a measure of labour progress: a longitudinal study." *BMC Pregnancy and Childbirth*. 2010.
http://www.biomedcentral.com/content/pdf/1471-2393-10-54.pdf

Nguyen, T.H., Larsen, T., Engholm, G., & Møller, H. "Evaluation of ultrasound-estimated date of delivery in 17,450 spontaneous singleton births: Do we need to modify Naegele's rule?" *Ultrasound Obstet Gynecol*. 1999 Jul;14(1):23–8.

European Society of Human Reproduction and Embryology. "Length of human pregnancies can vary naturally by as much as 5 weeks." August 2013.
http://www.eurekalert.org/pub_releases/2013-08/esoh-loh080513.php

Thacker, Stephen, & Stroup, Donna. "Revisiting the use of the electronic fetal monitor. *The Lancet,* 2003. 361, 445–446.
http://midwiferyservices.org/Revisiting%20the%20use%20of%20the%20
electronic%20fetal%20monitor.pdf

Thacker, Stephen, Stroup, D. "Continuous electronic heart rate monitoring for fetal assessment during labor." *CDEC.* 2000.
http://www.ncbi.nlm.nih.gov/pubmed/10796109

Childbirth.org. What is fetal monitoring?
http://www.childbirth.org/articles/efmfaq.html

Dr. H., Kieler, O. Axelsson, S. Nilsson, U. Waldenströ. "The length of human pregnancy as calculated by ultrasonographic measurement of the fetal biparietal diameter." *Ultrasound in Obstetrics and Gynecology.* Jan. 2003.
http://onlinelibrary.wiley.com/doi/10.1046/j.1469-0705.1995.06050353.x/abstract

Errol R., MD, PhD, Charles J. Lockwood, MD, Vanessa A Barss, MD. "Postterm Pregnancy."
http://www.uptodate.com/contents/postterm-pregnancy. UptoDate.com Sept 2013.

Mannino F., Neonatal complications of post-term gestation. *J Reprod Med.* Department of Pediatrics, University of California, San Diego. 1988 Mar;33(3):271–6.
http://www.ncbi.nlm.nih.gov/pubmed/3361517

The WHO Fortaleza, Brazil, April, 1985 and the "Summary Report" of The WHO Consensus Conference on Appropriate Technology Following Birth Trieste, October, 1986.

Study Finds Adverse Effects of Pitocin in Newborns. ACOG. May 2013.

"Study Links Inducing/Augmenting Labor with Modestly Higher Autism Risk." *Autism Speaks.* August 2013
http://www.autismspeaks.org/science/science-news/study-links-inducing
augmenting-labor-modestly-higher-autism-risk

Turner, R.A., Altemus, M., Enos, T., Cooper, B., & McGuinness, T. Preliminary research on plasma oxytocin in normal cycling women: investigating emotion and interpersonal distress. California School of Professional Psychology, San Francisco, USAPsychiatry 1999.
http://www.ncbi.nlm.nih.gov/pubmed/10420425

Lewis, Megan J., "An Investigation of the Effects of Pitocin for Labor." *Induction and Augmentation on Breastfeeding.* Scripps College. April 2012.

Uptodate.com. Pitocin. Cervidil. Cytotec: Drug Information.

"Meconium Aspiration." *Medline Plus.* 2011.

Cohain Slome, Judy. "The Epidural Trip. Why are so many women taking dangerous drugs during labor?" *Midwifery Today.* 2010.

Dunn, Peter. "Dr. Grantley Dick-Read of Norfolk and natural childbirth." Perinatal Lessons from the Past. *Arch Dis Child Fetal Neonatal Ed.* 1994.
http://www.ncbi.nlm.nih.gov/pmc/articles/PMC1061103/pdf/archdischfn00037-0073.pdf

Buckley, MD. Sarah. Epidurals: Risks and Concerns for Mother and Baby. *Gentle Birth, Gentle Mothering,* (Celestial Arts 2009).

Sandelowski, Margarete. Book Review. "Pain, pleasure, and American childbirth. From the Twilight Sleep to the Read Method," 1914–1960. U.S. National Library of Medicine. National Institutes of Health. 1986.
http://www.ncbi.nlm.nih.gov/pmc/articles/PMC1139622/?page=1

Kathryn Leggitt, RNC, MS, CNM. "How Has Childbirth Changed in This Century? University of Minnesota.
http://www.takingcharge.csh.umn.edu/explore-healing-practices/holistic-pregnancy-childbirth/how-has-childbirth-changed-century

Epidural Anesthesia. American Pregnancy Association.
http://americanpregnancy.org/labornbirth/epidural.html

VBAC or Repeat C-Section. Childbirthconnection.com
http://www.childbirthconnection.org/article.asp?ck=10214

Boyle, A. Reddy UM. Primary Cesarean Delivery in the United States. Obstetrics Gynecology. Dept of Obstetrics and Gynecology. July 2013.
http://www.ncbi.nlm.nih.gov/pubmed/23743454

Cesarean Section—A Brief History. NIH, US National Library of Medicine
http://www.nlm.nih.gov/exhibition/cesarean/part1.html

American Pregnancy Association. Cesarean Sections

University of Maryland Medical Center. C-section series. 2013.
http://umm.edu/health/medical/pregnancy/labor-and-delivery/csection-series

Chapter 4—The Emotions of Pregnancy and Birth

Bruggemann, Odalea, & Parpinelli, Mary. "Support to woman by a companion of her choice during childbirth: a randomized controlled trial." *Reproductive Health*, 2007. http://www.reproductive-health-journal.com/content/4/1/5

Larimore, W.L. "The Role of the Father in Childbirth." *Midwifery Today*. Issue No. 51, Autumn, 1999.

Odent, M. Is the Participation of the Father at Birth Dangerous? *Midwifery Today*. 1999.

LifeNew.com Aborting People With Down Syndrome: No Such Thing as a Life Not Worth Living

What is Birth Trauma? Birth Trauma Association.

What is Post-Traumatic Stress Disorder (PTSD)? National Institute of Mental Health.

Lusskin, Shari I., MD, FAPA Shaila Misri, MD, FRCPC. "Postpartum Blues and Depression." UptoDate.com 2013.

The Fertility Awareness Network. P.O. Box 1190, New York, NY 10009; (212) 475-4490. www.FertAware.com.

FDA. Mirena. FAERS. http://media2.newsnet5.com/uploads/WEWSMirenaDetailedReport.pdf

Hilgers, Thomas W. "The intrauterine device: contraceptive or abortifacient?" "Minnesota Medicine," June, 1974, 493-501.

Tarun Jain, MD & Ilana B. Ressler, MD. "Reversible contraception: Does it affect future fertility?" *Contemporary OB/Gyn*. SEP 2010. http://contemporaryobgyn.modernmedicine.com/contemporary-obgyn/news/modernmedicine/modern-medicine-now/reversible-contraception-does-it-affect-f

Mayo Clinic "Choosing a Birth Control Pill." http://www.mayoclinic.com/health/best-birth-control-pill/MY00996 *Mayo Clin Proc.* 2006 Oct;81(10):1290–302.

Kahlenborn, C., Modugno, F., Potter, D.M., & Severs, W.B. "Oral contraceptive use as a risk factor for premenopausal breast cancer: A meta-analysis." Department of Internal Medicine, Altoona Hospital, Altoona, PA. http://www.ncbi.nlm.nih.gov/pubmed/17036554

Polycarp research institute.
http://polycarp.org/statement_mayo_clinic_article.htm

Chapter 5—Guide to Common Pregnancy Conditions and Childbirth Treatments

MacRepertory and *Reference Works*. Homeopathic library software by Synergy, formerly known as Kent Homeopathic Associates.

Homeopathic Medicines for Pregnancy and Childbirth, by Richard Moskowitz, M.D. (North Atlantic Books. 1992)

Homeopathy for Pregnancy, Birth, and Your Baby's First Year, by Miranda Castro (Macmillan London Ltd. 1993)

Homeopathy for the Modern Pregnant Woman and Her Infant: A Therapeutic Practice Guidebook for Midwives, Physicians and Practitioners, by Sandra J. Perko (Benchmark Homeopathic Publications 1997).

Ina May's Guide to Childbirth, by Ina May Gaskin (Bantam Books, 2003)

Myofunctional Therapy
http://www.joymoeller.com

Natural Baby and Childcare, by Lauren Feder, M.D. (Hatherleigh Press. 2006)

Tongue Tie: From Confusion to Clarity http://www.tonguetie.net